Forty Days of Yoga

Breaking down the barriers to a home yoga practice

"There is an esoteric secret to Yoga to receive its many wonderful gifts. You already do Yoga! You practice in the way that is right for you – actually, naturally and non obsessively until there is no issue. It's just like brushing your teeth or taking a shower – daily and no big deal. Yet we have an inbuilt resistance to practicing and overcoming obstacles to life. Please read Kara-Leah's book because she will help you through this and initiate you into daily practice. You will become a Yogi and dive deep into your intimate life in every way."

Mark Whitwell author, *Yoga of Heart* and *The Promise of Love, Sex, and Intimacy*, USA

"Forty Days of Yoga is absolutely brilliant. It is a powerful crystalizing of Kara-Leah's accumulated experience of flourishing her own practice in the reality of day-to-day life, complete with so many of the common challenges. The worksheets are a fantastic way for readers to put the wisdom shared in the narrative of the book into immediate action. I love that the whole reading experience feels just like sitting down to a cup of tea with KL. And that is a treat indeed!"

Kelly Fisher, Director of Urban Yoga, Wellington, New Zealand

"I've felt frustrated trying to find the right classes, times, and locations to keep yoga in my schedule. And most home yoga instruction is over-simplified, disconnected 'watch this video and follow along.' Kara-Leah takes you so much deeper, guiding you into a home yoga practice that is alive with customization and creativity. This is much more than a reference book about poses or a personal development pep-talk. If you're attempting to do yoga at home, this is a fantastic set of tools."

Slade Roberson, intuitive counselor and author of *Shift Your Spirits*, USA

"Forty Days of Yoga is a powerful resource for anyone interested in committing to a home yoga practice. Drawing from her years of experience, Kara-Leah beautifully shines a light on all the myriad obstacles, internal and external, that one can face when undertaking a self-directed practice while living an ordinary life in the world. Packed full of ingeniously practical worksheets and examples from Kara-Leah's own life, this book invites one inwards to reflect honestly and creatively on one's own process and aspirations. And it is all done in a wonderfully holistic, all-inclusive way, so that one's whole life becomes part of the solution, rather than being seen as a 'problem'. I highly recommend this beautiful book!"

Peter Fernando, Insight meditation teacher and creator of A Month of Mindfulness online course, Wellington, New Zealand

"From the first page, I was hooked. It's not about what you practice, it's not about which poses you do or if you can touch your knee with your nose in a forward bend. None of that matters. What matters is that you turn up to the mat every day and do a mindful yoga practice of some description. If you want a home practice, but for reasons known and unknown you have not been able to do it, I suggest you invest in this book. Truly, it's a life changer."

Sara Foley, Freelance Writer & Blogger, Smells Good, Feels Good, Australia

"Knowing Kara-Leah's Musings from the Mat column, I didn't even pause before considering downloading Forty Days of Yoga. Such a happy surprise to find it stays away from prescriptions of yoga poses but instead fills my practice with questions that have me thinking, and meanings that add substance. It is a truly enriching book."

Cate Peterson, founder of YogaPass, Australia

Forty Days
of Yoga

Breaking down the barriers
to a home yoga practice

by Kara-Leah Grant

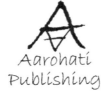

Aarohati
Publishing

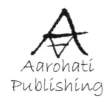

Aarohati
Publishing

P.O. Box 108

Glenorchy, New Zealand

Copyright © Kara-Leah Grant 2013

First published March 2013

Book design: Kara-Leah Grant

Photography: Michael Hobbs

ISBN: 978-0-473-23958-9

Contents Page

Introduction

More than ten years after I started practicing yoga and eight years after I started a home yoga practice, I still struggle to turn up to the mat daily.

It's not because I don't know what to do – I'm a yoga teacher. I know what to do.

It's not because I don't have enough time, or the right space, or a supporting environment. I have all of those things, and it still takes effort and determination to practice daily.

I know the same is true for you. You want to practice yoga at home.

But you don't. Or you do, but then you stop.

You may think it's because you don't know what to do. You may think it's because you don't have time or space or support.

It's none of those things. It's... something else.

It's the mind, getting in the way.

I know this, because over the last ten years or so, I've been committed to practicing yoga. Not always by choice – but because it was necessary for my physical, mental and emotional well-being.

When I was 16 years old, my spine was fused at L4/5. My back felt great for a few years, but I never addressed the underlying causes of my spinal issues and by the time I was 25, I was in daily pain. I had excruciating sciatic pain down my right leg and my right foot was half numb. My situation had become so dire I was walking with a limp. I was facing a painful future with limited mobility and possibly more surgery.

I'd tried yoga four years previously – a ten-week Iyengar course. Travels and life had since intervened, but somehow I knew that yoga was the one thing that could help me heal my body.

I was right. Yoga classes made a world of difference and I was on my way back to physical health.

Four years after that decision to make yoga a part of my life, I had two psychotic episodes a month apart. Triggered by a combination of drug use (LSD), relationship difficulties and life stresses, these psychotic episodes also broke my mind wide open. I experienced Bliss – and a shocking comedown.

Nothing could ever be the same after that. This time it was my mental and emotional self that needed yoga – and not just classes, but a regular home practice. That was the beginning of my home practice. It wasn't something I started for fun, or because I wanted it even. No, I started my home practice because I desperately needed the small moments of peace it brought me on my mat. I needed my home practice to help me pick up the broken parts of psyche and put them back together again.

In the nine years since those two episodes of psychosis I persisted with my practice – no matter what obstacles arose –because of the enormous difference my practice made to my physical, mental and emotional well-being. Without yoga, life became a struggle and I could barely keep my head above water. With yoga, I was able to systematically work through the many challenges that came my way.

I learned, through application and practice, that the only thing ever standing between me and my practice was my mind.

The same is true for you.

The only thing ever standing between you and your practice is your mind.

In this book we're going to examine that mind of yours and all the ways it can sabotage even the very best of intentions.

That means that if you're looking for a home yoga practice book that will tell you *what* to do, this is not it. I don't tell you how to do any postures at all, there's no instructions on pranayama and I don't talk about how to meditate. There's a myriad of other sources you can find for that kind of information (see the back of the book for a list of resources I use and love).

What you can't get anywhere else is my detailed process for deconstructing the many obstacles that prevent us from practicing.

Like yoga itself, this book is about the process – the process that will carry you to, and through, *Forty Days of Yoga.*

I know – you're looking for a magic bullet. That perfect home yoga practice that will turn you into a yogi. I know this because at workshops and in classes, via email and feedback, student after student after student asks me, and other teachers:

'What's your home practice like?'

Students have this idea that there is an ideal home yoga practice, and if they could just find out what it is, they'd be able to practice it and all would be well. Hopefully this ideal home yoga practice would be short-ish, easy-ish and work miracles on the body, mind and soul.

But you know what? There is no standardized ideal home yoga practice. There is only *your* ideal home yoga practice. What that is depends on many factors, including your body, your stage of life, your living environment, your work environment, your culture, your climate... your *everything.*

That's why I can't tell you what to do. But I can take you through a process that unlocks your own desire and ability to discover your ideal home yoga practice.

What does it mean to practice at home every day?

It means you move, mindfully.

It means you breathe, mindfully.

It means you simply *be*, mindfully.

You move, breathe, and be in your life.

The *what* of practice ceases to be important, as the *how* supersedes everything else. Because the how is the Yoga. More on that later.

This book won't be easy though. It's going to make demands.

It will demand that you stop reading, pick up a pen and write. It will demand that you dig deep into your psyche to get to the truth of your motivations and intentions for a home yoga practice. This book will demand that you take an honest look at your life and the people in it to see who supports your yoga practice and who doesn't. It will demand that you make changes, of your own choosing, but changes nonetheless.

If you're not up for this – if you're not ready to take action, you might as well stop reading right now. Give this book to someone else. Because it won't help you. Instead it will only be another distraction, another thing separating you out from life, and from Yoga.

But if you're up for the challenge, if you want to experience a changed life, and a changed way of seeing life, then keep reading. This book will give you everything you need to commit to *Forty Days of Yoga* and stick to it.

Gather a pen and a notebook – something you can use to record your experience of this book and complete the worksheets, and something you can add to over time – as you track your practice.

Together, we'll make a yogi of you yet!

How to use this workbook:

How you use this workbook is up to you.

You may read it through from beginning to end and then go back and do the worksheets. You may stop at each worksheet and do the exercises immediately, taking time to consider the implications of each process.

All the worksheets have been included at the end of the book so you can fill in your answers. Or you may wish to use a journal or loose leaf paper in your own binder. You may even wish to create a file on your computer.

The trick to the worksheets is to work fast, getting past the internal censor. Don't think about answers, just start writing whatever comes to mind, no matter how 'right' you think it is, or how silly it sounds.

If you feel resistance arising to anything, notice it. Breathe into it, and give yourself a pep talk. Something simple like,

> *'I want to easily complete these worksheets because it's going to help me commit to a home yoga practice.'*

In this way, the process of reading the book and filling in the worksheets becomes your yoga.

The final chapters of the book look at on what happens once you start practicing. It is useful to read through these chapters before you start your *Forty Days of Yoga* so that when things happens on the mat, or even before you get on your mat, you remember.

'A-ha! This was mentioned in the book!'

Finally, the book has been written as a reference. It's something you can return to again and again throughout your practice.

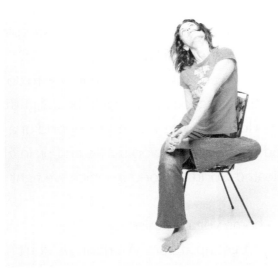

Yoga moves us from the inside out, a dance with breath and life

What is a Home Yoga Practice?

We all have ideas about what it means to practice yoga at home.

Often those ideas revolve around getting up at 5am, rolling out the mat in a special space reserved for practicing yoga, preferably overlooking a forest, mountain or ocean view, and stepping on our mats to do a thorough 90 minute practice encompassing asana, pranayama and meditation.

That's what a home yoga practice is right?

But what if it isn't?

What if those ideas of what a home yoga practice is are stopping you from creating, committing and sticking to your Ideal Home Yoga Practice?

In an ideal world, getting up at 5am and taking ninety minutes to do our practice, un-interrupted and peaceful, with a gorgeous view would be delightful. But this is not an ideal world. It's a real world. For most of us, it's the world of a householder with children and partners and flatmates and workmates and plain old mates. It's a busy world and it's a complicated world. A world in which we fight for time and space to call our own.

This ideal concept of what a home yoga practice is can limit us, stall us, and set us up for failure. We think we can't get up at 5am. We think we don't have the right space. We think we can't do 90 minutes. We think we don't know what to do.

What if a home yoga practice is something different?

What if we broadened our perspective and stepped away from limiting ideas of space, time, and action?

What if a home yoga practice was nothing more than something we do by ourselves that connects us to something greater than ourselves.

What then?

Let's step back a moment. If you're reading this book, you probably practice yoga in some way, shape or form, and it's likely you've heard many definitions of yoga.

Maybe you think yoga is postures. Maybe you think yoga means to join together, or union. Maybe you think it's using the breath to link the mind to the body.

Yoga is all those things and more.

When we practice yoga – when we're on a path of yoga – we're shifting our sense of identity from the small limited ego mind self to a larger, connected, Divine sense of Self that yogis call the Atman.

That's what Yoga is – a path from small self to Big Self. When you experience that sense of Big Self you realise that it's not so much a sense of identity as a state of being.

But don't take my word for it. Through your practice, find out for yourself. Yoga is experiential – you experience it to know it.

Until you do experience Yoga as a state of being, bear these things in mind...

First, Yoga is a *path* to self-realisation (realising the different, larger, connected, divine sense of Self). It's also the *destination* at the end of that path – at its essence a state of being.

The paradox is that state of being isn't something far off in the future that we attain after years and years of practice.

That state of being is available right here, right now, in every moment. It's when we're present – truly present to all that is. It's when we're able to accept what is arising in the moment and stay with all the feelings and sensations in our bodies. And it's when we're able to observe our mind and know we are not our thoughts.

So Yoga is a *path* to self-realisation and it is also that *state of being* we experience when we're self-realised.

Yoga – with a capital Y – is *both* the path and the destination.

One merges into the other.

Finally, yoga (with a small y) is the *practice* we do along the path to our destination.

We *practice* shifting from small self (ego/mind) to Big Self (Atman) by using specific tools and techniques like asana, pranayama, meditation, chanting, and visualisation.

What tools we use to practice shifting states of being are not important – only that they serve us. *The 'what' is not the Yoga.* It's just a tool or a technique.

Asana is not yoga – it's a tool we use to *practice* on our path of Yoga to our destination of Yoga.

When we arrive, there is nowhere to go. Practicing along the path of yoga has merged us *into* Yoga.

The beauty of perceiving our practice in this way is that suddenly *everything* in our life can be Yoga. It's how we parent. How we work. How we love. How we learn. How we live.

This is how Yoga has always been and it's why there are four major yoga paths or four different ways to walk the yogic path.

Our yoga path can be through love (Bhakti Yoga), through work (Karma Yoga), through knowledge (Jnana Yoga) or through our mind/bodies (Raja Yoga).

This is not an either/or equation. While most of us have a natural tendency towards one path or another, many of us will walk more than one yoga path in our lifetime.

Raja Yoga, out of which springs Hatha Yoga, has been further conceptualised by Patanjali, an early yogi and author of the *Yoga Sutras*, into eight limbs:

> *Yamas* – Ways to behave towards others including non-violence, truth, non-stealing, non-accumulation and walking with Higher Self
>
> *Niyamas* – Ways to behave towards the Self including purity, contentment, burning through impurities, study and surrender
>
> *Asana* – Physical postures
>
> *Pranayama* – Breath work
>
> *Pratyahara* – Withdrawal of the senses
>
> *Dharana* – Concentration
>
> *Dhyana* – Meditation
>
> *Samadhi* – Bliss, or Super-consciousness

We're not going in-depth into each of these limbs – suffice to say
sequential: they happen concurrently with each other. Most western
onto the yogic path through the practice of asana, but it is only one aspect o
path.

Knowing these – the many paths of Yoga – helps us to understand that our
home yoga practice is not limited to asana, or posture. That is only one aspect
of the path of Raja Yoga and it is not the only path there is. However, it is the
path that most Westeners need the most. We live in our heads, our bodies are
tight and stiff and shut-down, and before we can open to other ways of seeing
life, we have to open our bodies. Before we can sit comfortably for meditation,
pranayama or chanting, we need to open and free our bodies. Before we can still
our minds enough for meditation, it helps to practice asana.

Mostly, in this book, I will be assuming that you're starting with a physical
practice. However, I'm *also* assuming this physical practice could include
pranayama, meditation, chanting, mudra and visualisation.

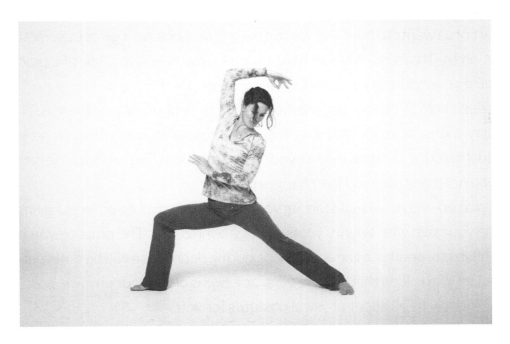

Yoga moves us from our heads, down into our bodies.

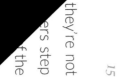

if you want to start a home yoga practice, while your
more ease in the body, mind or emotions, on a deeper
nat dedicating one's life to Yoga is dedicating one's life
; one's life to realising the Self.

e're not just here to discipline ourselves into moving
understand ourselves *through* moving our body every
day.

We commit to stepping on to the path, day after day. We practice the tools and techniques of Yoga. Eventually that state of being we practice on the path grows and expands until we notice it seeping out and into our entire life.

We have begun to realise the Self.

It might take years or decades before that happens, and in the meantime we step back onto the path day after day, practicing our Yoga, whatever it might be.

There is great freedom in knowing that *what* we do in our yoga practice doesn't matter.

Only that we do it.

Yet great freedom can also be terrifying.

A part of us wants to have this *specific thing to do*, because it gives us something to hold on to. That's ok. You can have that too. You can have a specific practice that you do every single day, if that's what you need.

But don't hold tightly to that practice as if it's the only right way there is. There are many paths, as many paths as there are people to walk them. Yoga is an individual practice, designed to suit your needs and your lifestyle. Like everything, what you need and how you live changes constantly.

The practice you have as a starting yogi aged twenty will be different from the practice you have with twenty years of yoga behind you. The practice you have after childbirth, or after a car accident, or during depression will be different.

So let go of the idea that a home yoga practice is only about physical postures, although it may be all about physical postures for you.

Let go of the idea that it has to be at least ninety minutes, or an hour, or thirty minutes to be 'worth it' and 'good'.

Let go of the idea that you have to know what you're doing.

This is where our home yoga practice begins.

With a clean slate.

An empty mind.

Beginner's mind.

An understanding that *how* we do *what* we do is all that matters.

A home yoga practice? Nothing more than a path home to a deeper sense of being.

The Difference between a Home Practice and Class

A home yoga practice is different from going to classes, workshops and retreats.

Why? Because when we practice yoga on our own, we're forced to tune in and connect to our own inner teacher. We're forced to rely on ourselves and, over time, we learn what it is that we need to do.

Because that's the thing – yoga is a personal practice. It's not meant to be experienced in large classes day after day, week after week. Yoga is something personal that you do by yourself, and you do what it is that you need. That's not always possible in a class situation.

Classes are valuable – they're a wonderful way to learn the tools of yoga – the specific postures and techniques we use to come into that state of being called Yoga. Going to class makes us feel connected to a community and it gives us the opportunity to work with an external teacher.

But it doesn't give us that 100% connection to our own inner teacher and the ability to trust where our internal teacher is going to guide us.

When we go to class, we hand over responsibility for our practice, and to some extent our body, to another person. In class we are implicitly saying,

'You tell me what to do. You tell me what's best for me.'

Plus a class will never give us the exact yoga practice we need because a yoga teacher can't possibly instruct a class to take account of everyone's physical, emotional, mental and spiritual needs.

At some point on our yoga journey – possibly now, given you're reading this book – we find we're ready to take responsibility for our own practice.

There are also practical reasons for starting a home yoga practice. Sometimes it's not that we're ready to deepen our practice at all, but that we don't have any choice. Maybe we live a long way from classes. Maybe we can't afford to go to class. Maybe we don't connect with any of the teachers in our area.

We may have specific needs in our yoga practice. We're experiencing some kind of mental anguish or illness, or our bodies have limitations that need individual attention, or we have a disability, or are recovering from a serious illness. A regular yoga class aimed at the able-bodied doesn't work for us. The right home practice can greatly improve our quality of life.

It doesn't matter why we take the leap into home practice, only that we do. A home yoga practice is a necessity if you really want to walk that path to Self. No one else can walk with you. That's when you make the leap from being a yoga student to being a yogi.

That doesn't mean you can't continue going to class once you start a home yoga practice. In fact, having a daily practice and including a class or two a week can be a crucial way to get external feedback on what you're doing. It's an excellent way to learn new tools and techniques, and continue to feel a part of your community. However if you've committed to a daily practice, going to class doesn't count as your practice for that day.

If you go to class, and take fifteen minutes in the yoga room before class, tuning in and practicing... well you could count that as a home yoga practice. If you really had to. But let's not nitpick here.

Class teaches technique and tools, and can show us our blind spots.

Home practice teaches empowerment, self-reliance and deepens our connection to Self.

Yoga students go to class

Yogis practice at home (as well as attend class).

An exceptional yoga teacher will create an atmosphere in class that allows each student to find their own way to yoga, and these are the classes and teachers to seek out. Exceptional teachers will also encourage you to start practicing yoga at home. If possible, these are the classes you want to attend, as they will support you in your home practice journey.

When we practice at home we're alone. It's just you and your breath. You and your body. You and your mind. How many of us ever do that?

Even when we go to the gym or for a run, we're reading a magazine, we're watching TV, we're listening to music. We're doing whatever we can to distract ourselves from where we are and what we're doing. At home, we're with friends, family, facebook, TV, on the phone, on the Internet, always *on*, always *with*, always *doing*.

Yoga is where all of that stops.

No more distraction.

Just you.

That's one reason why we resist and procrastinate and do everything we can to avoid starting or maintaining a home yoga practice: because we know in our heart of hearts we will have to face ourselves.

That can be scary.

None of us admit the whole truth about ourselves, even to ourselves. We hide things away, tuck them out of sight, shielding and contracting ourselves against ourselves. All this denial, hiding and shielding happens in our bodies and in our mind – the very things we must be fully present with when we practice yoga.

Coming to our mat, by ourselves, can be the first time we ever begin to look at ourselves. We don't always like what we see. We don't want to see it. We don't want to know.

Let me tell you a story:

The first ten years of my practice, particularly my home practice and Bikram classes, were marked by deep sobbing despair. Not every class. Not all the time. Not the entire class. But enough.

At first I assumed it was the unexpressed heartache at the ending of a recent relationship. But as the tears continued, it had to be more. I realised it was the unexpressed tears of a lifetime of emotional suppression. Even those tears had to have an ending, yet still I cried. Tears and tears and tears and tears.

In class, the tears were bearable. Postures kept me distracted. The teacher kept me distracted. I could weep, silently, while continuing on, skating along the surface of those tears.

At home, I dreaded getting on my mat. Some days it felt like the air between my mat and I thickened until I had to will myself to press through it and down into Child's Pose. Those days were the days when I cried the most. Often I never made it past that first Child Pose. I lay and I sobbed and I broke through the ice that had kept me, my body and my mind frozen in time for so long.

One day, it stopped.

I don't remember what day.

I only know that I don't cry on the mat anymore. Not unless there's something specific in my life to cry about. No more old tears. No more world tears.

If I hadn't had a home practice, I doubt I would ever have allowed myself to sink beneath the surface of all those tears. The only reason I was so committed to my home practice was because I was teaching yoga. If I was teaching, I had to get on my mat every day, even when that wall of resistance threatened to beat me back, because I was a teacher and that's what teachers have to do. My commitment to my students was greater than my commitment to myself.

Your yoga journey will be different from mine.

Your home practice will be different from mine.

But your commitment must be the same:

> *No matter what, get on your mat.*
> *No matter what, stay with what arises.*
> *No matter what, keep coming back.*

Have the courage to face yourself – all of yourself.

For if you can't face yourself, how will you ever face the world? And if you can't face yourself, how can you expect anyone else to?

Yoga strips us bare – all illusions, all walls, all masks. Gone.

That is freedom.

To no longer have to pretend, or hide, or hold up the wall.

You won't get that from class. That's why home yoga practice is essential if you want to shift from being a student to being a yogi. And you do, right? That's why you're reading this book.

Teaching and Practicing Yoga ~ What's The Difference?

For those of us who teach yoga, we spend so much time teaching or prepping for class, our own practice sometimes goes out the window.

All the work around preparing for class – sequencing, practicing the class, creating playlists, learning sequences – means we have less time than ever and it's easy to let our own practice go because we reason that we're still 'practicing yoga' when we teach.

That's plenty of practice of asana... right?

Yes... but practice of asana while your attention is focused on the external – students and the class – is not a home yoga practice.

You're not tuning into your own wisdom and sitting with what arises within your own body. There's a lack of depth, or connection. Or maybe just a different kind of depth and connection when you teach as opposed to when you practice.

Regardless, teaching and a home practice are two different experiences.

Once you start teaching, it's more important than ever to maintain a consistent, dedicated daily practice. That time of connecting to source feeds you and it feeds your teaching. It's filling the well so you've got something to offer when you're in front of a class. Let that practice go and you'll have less and less to draw from.

However, what your home yoga practice looks like, as a teacher, can shift and change. First, let's define what it is a teacher does:

- Teaching class, including demonstrating
- Prepping for class, including putting together and practicing sequences, exploring and playing with specific asana
- Home practice

These are three different experiences.

-Teaching is mostly external. Prepping is both internal and external, and practice is all internal. It can be tempting to classify prepping as practice, but it's not the same thing.

When you prep for class, you are focusing on the needs of the class you're teaching – you're choosing, exploring and playing with the appropriate asana and sequences for the class.

When you first start teaching the demands and needs of your classes will often overlap with your own demands and needs for practice. Over time, as you deepen your practice, what you teach, and what you need to practice may shift further and further apart.

A deepening practice doesn't have to mean doing more and more complicated asana, but that you are venturing deeper and deeper into those asana, or adding more pranayama, meditation or other aspects of yoga like chanting.

If you rely on your prep as your practice, you won't be meeting your own needs as a teacher and you will burn out.

Make sure that you maintain a balance of teaching, prepping and practice. Allow your practice to shift and change to meet your needs. It might include reading from yogic texts, more meditation, pranayama, chanting. You might practice less asana in a session, but go longer and deeper into those asana so further nuances reveal themselves.

If you're teaching a set sequence like Bikram, and attending classes at the studio you teach in, that doesn't count as a home yoga practice. But your home practice doesn't mean doing ninety minutes of Bikram every day. It might mean ten minutes of meditation. It might mean reading yogic texts. It might mean pranayama. It might mean taking one asana and playing with it for ten minutes. Bikram teachers can have a home practice too!

If you're teaching Astanga, the home practice is defined. You know exactly what you're doing, and there is no question about it.

That doesn't mean you can't *also* take some time to explore each posture on its own, taking ten or more minutes to breathe your way into it, and seeing how different that asana is when it's not sandwiched between two other postures and only held for five breaths.

If you're a yoga teacher, getting clear about what you need in a home yoga practice is even more important, as is sticking to it. You owe it to yourself, and you owe it to your students.

The Evolution of a Home Yoga Practice

Like anything, a home yoga practice will change over time.

When we begin, our biggest concern is:

'What am I going to do?'

As a beginning home practitioner, it makes sense to have a concrete and specific idea of exactly what you're going to do, so you can focus on doing it. Getting on the mat and getting lost can feel like a waste of time. You can spend all your time wondering:

'Am I doing this right?
What comes next?
Where does this leg go again?'

All of these questions take us out of our practice.

Over years of practice – yes years! – what we're doing will evolve. Instead of working with a specific set of postures, we'll know enough to vary our practice. Sometimes we'll vary it because of the moon cycle, or the seasons. Sometimes we'll vary it so we work through a complete range of movements over a week or a month.

Eventually, we'll become more sensitive to our bodies, minds and emotional state. As this happens, we'll be able to intuit the practice we need to support ourselves through whatever state we're in. On days when we're exhausted, we'll naturally feel the need for a restorative practice and will have built up enough sensitivity and confidence to know how to do this.

Finally, our practice may evolve to the point where we're able to discern the movement of Prana (life-force) in the body and surrender to its flow, allowing it to lead us through our practice. For some people, this won't happen: not in this lifetime anyway. For other people, it may happen a year into practice.

It doesn't matter. These stages are not levels, nor is one more important than the other. We're not trying to graduate or move from one stage to the next. All we need to do is be aware of what our needs are and what stage we're at – and allow our practice to reflect that. Otherwise, we'll get frustrated and worn out and feel like we're failing at our practice.

These stages also reflect the slow shift from a mostly asana-based practice to a mostly-meditative practice. Sometimes these changes can also reflect our age. Our practice can shift as we get older – although there is no need to stop doing asana just because you've had another birthday. Yoga teachers are famed for continuing on just as they always have right into their 90s.

Knowing this natural evolution helps us to stick with our practice through our life transitions and through the tough times.

I'm making up this 'evolution scale'. It's just a conceptual model to guide you to the right place for you. Hold to it lightly!

Evolution of a Home Yoga Practice Scale					
	Beginner	**Beginner / Intermediate**	**Intermediate**	**Experienced / Intermediate**	**Experienced**
Practice History	Never practiced at home before	Has done a small amount of home practice	Has had a consistent home practice for short time	Has practiced at home for a couple of years	Five or more years of home practice
Type of Practice Suggested	Structured	Structured	Structured with some exploration	Exploration	Breath or Prana-led

Where do you see yourself on this scale?

Beside how long you've been practicing, there are other variables which will influence where you fall on this scale.

For example:

> If you've done other mind-body practices like Tai Chi or Karate, or even Pilates, that can give you more body awareness or energy awareness.
>
> If you're highly intuitive, such as a practicing psychic or energy worker, this can also mean you're more tuned into energy.

In these cases, while you may not have had much actual yoga practice, you may still have a refined ability to work with your body.

Your ideal home practice might be more structured, with some exploration, or even with strong parameters.

The scale is a guide only, and you will need to assess where you sit on it.

Figuring out where you sit on this scale helps you determine what kind of practice you need. Working with where you are, and giving yourself what you need is really important. It helps you to stay on track.

It doesn't matter where you are on the scale. It's not a good/bad kind of scale, nor a better/worse. Some people spend their entire life in a structured practice because that's perfect for them, and always will be. You're not trying to get from one end of the scale to the other.

Success lies in being in the perfect place for you. Wherever you are.

As beginning yogis, our practice demands that we open up to receive information, as Yoga is a completely different way of seeing the world for many people.

There is so much to take in – a different language, philosophy, postures, breath, styles, paths... it is easy at the beginning to be overwhelmed

So keep it simple. Beginning with a simple asana sequence is enough. Learn this deeply. Stay with this until something within you – deep within you, not a bored monkey-mind seeking the next distraction – feels compelled to seek out the next piece of the puzzle. Take that piece and practice it. Explore it, play with it, integrate it and wait again until the inner yearning grows strong for the next piece and the next piece and the next piece.

Most of all, do your practice. It will lead you.

As Sri. K Pattabhi Jois famously said;

'Do your practice and all is coming'.

This is a gentle reminder that no questions are needed. That no teacher is even needed. That when you do your practice, day in and day out, whatever that practice may be and however that practice may shift and change, the next piece of the puzzle will arise and appear when you are ready. You will know what to do or how to find out what to do. Everything is perfect, in sequence and happening just as it needs to. Provided you show up and do your practice.

If you don't practice... that too is perfect. It's just where you are right now. Until you aren't anymore and you're practicing again.

This evolution of practice also points to the great difference between going to class and doing your home yoga practice.

In one, you seek answers externally and the exceptional teachers gently guide you back to yourself to find the answers.

In the other, you seek answers internally. Out of this internal seeking arises a knowing that all we ever need resides inside of us. With that knowing, all our insecurities and fears drop away. We have arrived, to where we always were.

So do your practice, as it evolves over time. All is coming.

Working with Parameters

Before we go on, more on parameters.

By now, you should have a clearer idea of where you sit on the Evolution of a Home Practice scale – whether you need more structure in your practice, or broad parameters or perhaps even an element of both of those.

If you suspect you're ready to work with parameters, or just want to know more about what it means to work with parameters, instead of a structured practice like Astanga, here's a run down.

We are creative beings, and we work well within parameters – whether they be of space, time, or something else like a specific body focus.

Like water needs a channel in which to flow, so too do we creative beings need parameters in which to practice. Otherwise we'll rock up to our mats ready to practice whatever it is we need to practice and...

We won't know what to do, or where to start.

Perfectly natural. Because you can't move into flow without moving into something. You have to start somewhere. It helps too if you've got somewhere to go. That's what I mean by parameters.

You can set all kinds of parameters, and it will depend on your reasons for practicing, and how far along the home yoga practice evolution you are.

A parameter might be time-based.

> *'I will practice for ten minutes, morning and evening.'*

It might be posture-based.

> *'I will do ten sun salutations every day, and end with a twist, backbend and Corpse Pose.'*

It might be kriya-based.

> *'I will do eleven minutes of this particular kriya.'*

It could be a combination.

> *'I will practice for twenty minutes, playing with sun salutations, Warrior variations and then a closing sequence.'*

Whatever it is, you know where you're starting, and the minimum amount of time you're going to practice. That's a parameter.

Even an unstructured home practice should have some kind of parameter to ground it, and you. Water needs a container or it bleeds out everywhere and evaporates. So does our practice. One minute it's there, the next minute it's been days and we haven't practiced. Parameters support us, and our practice.

The most basic parameter to work with is an understanding of structure, and no matter what you're doing – asana, pranayama, meditation, chanting or a combination – the basic structure is always the same.

Tune In

Warm Up

Sustain

Peak

Cool Down

Closing

For Example – Meditation:

Tune In – Take your seat, find breath connection, find your foundation, lengthen your spine.

Warm Up – Feel your breath, watch your mind, see where you are today, let yourself settle.

Sustain – Do the Practice.

Peak – Often the place where we find our greatest discomfort or challenge and want to stop. We have to keep coming back to our focus.

Cool down – Moving into the last few minutes of practice, perhaps releasing any tension in the legs or shifting position.

Close Your Practice – Take a moment to end, thank yourself for the practice, perhaps set an intention for the rest of the day.

For Example – Asana:

Tune In – Find breath connection, feel yourself in your body, find your foundation, lengthen or release, set an intention.

Warm Up – Sun salutations, cat/cow, any simple breath-led postures that move all parts of the body through a range of motion.

Sustain – Standing postures, into seated postures.

Peak – Usually the posture we've been working our practice toward. Sometimes a deep backbend, or an arm balance, or a deep hip-opener.

Cool down – Releasing any accumulated tension with counter-poses, backbend, twist, Corpse Pose.

Close Your Practice – Take a moment to end, thank yourself for the practice, perhaps set an intention for the rest of the day.

When you know a basic structure you don't have to know *exactly* what postures you're going to do – you can feel into it.

> *How do I tune in? Mountain pose, Child's pose, Easy Cross-Legged.*
> *How do I warm up? Sun salutations, Moon salutations.*
> *What can I do to sustain? Standing poses.*

It doesn't matter if postures don't perfectly sequence one after another, in time, you'll feel what works and what doesn't work, and intuitively know how to sequence. Like anything, it's just a learning process.

A parameter at its simplest, can just be a time factor.

> *'I'll practice for ten minutes a day.'*

It's also best if there is some rhyme or reason to the practice – it's not just whatever takes your fancy day by day. Asana one day, chanting the next, pranayama the day after.

Know that for forty days, you will meditate for ten minutes a day, and do body-opening asana for ten minutes.

That keeps you on track.

It's a delicate balance – moving away from structure and into parameters. You need to be discerning and alert to make sure at all times that it's not your state of mind leading your practice, but a deeper inner knowing of what's needed. Otherwise, you could be feeling lazy so decide to practice nothing but Corpse Pose. That's different from knowing you are exhausted and giving yourself the much-needed rest of Corpse Pose.

Whenever you doubt what's leading you, check in. Ask yourself:

> *Is it my fluctuating state of mind dictating my yoga practice right now?*
> *Or am I responding on a deeper level to what it is I need?*

You'll know.

The Magic of A Forty Day Practice

Committing to a life-long practice of yoga every single day for the rest of your life is daunting.

You. Must. Practice. Every. Day!

A sure way to fail if ever.

However, committing to practicing every single day for the next forty days is imminently doable. Forty days is just longer than a month and it's long enough to firmly ingrain a habit into our psyche.

There's also a mystical reverence with forty days – although no one can explain why forty days matters. All they can do is point towards Jesus' spending forty days in the desert arguing with the Devil (his shadow?), Noah's Ark floating for forty days, forty days of Lent and a host of other religious references to Forty Days.

The best reference I could come up with is that in yogic philosophy 'it's said' if you do something for forty days it becomes a habit. So let's go with that. (Who said it? Nobody knows...)

The beauty of committing for forty days is when you get to the end of the forty days you can decide to do another forty days and then another, and another. Each time you're recommitting and deepening the positive samskara of practicing yoga by yourself every single day.

(A samskara is an impression left in the psyche from an event, or what we do. Over time, like a wheel rut in mud, experiencing that same thing over and over leaves a deeper impression.)

Over time the practice of yoga becomes like eating, drinking, or even breathing. You love it, you see what it does for you, and you couldn't imagine not doing it every single day.

This is the process.

And it starts with *Forty Days of Yoga*. You can do that. You're going to do it. Look, you've done it!

When you begin the forty day process there is one rule and one rule only.

If you miss a day, the count starts again. This is crucial.

If you miss Day 36 you don't just continue on for four more days and say you've completed your *Forty Days of Yoga*. No, the next day, you start again at Day 1.

There's something interesting that happens in the mind when you do this. It means that next time you're tempted to skip a day or you've got a super busy day and contemplate letting the practice go, you remember it means you have to start again at Day 1.

No one likes to lose all the hard work they've accomplished and that extra motivation means you're less likely to skip a day. You're more likely to find a way to fit yoga into that super busy day.

Even if it means getting up twenty minutes earlier.

This is the magic of *Forty Days of Yoga*.

It's short enough to contemplate completing. It's long enough to build a habit. It's got historic and mystical relevance. Plus doing forty continuous days of yoga without skipping any days makes it important. It makes it a priority, something you care about and something that matters.

And that's what you want your Home Yoga Practice to be right? An important priority that you care about because it matters.

Time: How long is long enough?

One of the biggest stumbling blocks to creating and sticking to a home yoga practice is the idea that it must be a certain length – like ninety minutes – to have any value.

This is not true. According to yoga teacher and author Mark Whitwell, a home yoga practice can be as short as seven minutes a day.

Yes, seven minutes a day. That's how long it takes to connect to your breath and drop into the state of being that is Yoga.

It's also downright sneaky! When you get on your mat and do seven minutes, dropping into Yoga, you will find it difficult to get *off* your mat after those seven minutes. Likely you'll want to stay and often you will.

Seven minutes is how you fool your mind. It's how you get around all those other obstacles we'll investigate in the next chapter.

Anybody, no matter how busy they are, can find seven minutes in their day. *If you want to.*

Of course, the results you get if you spend seven minutes a day practicing are going to be different from the results you get from spending sixty minutes practicing or ninety minutes practicing... but not as different as you might imagine.

Yoga works on quality and depth, not on time.

In a short practice, knowing we've only got limited time, we'll often drop in faster and be more present with what we're doing because we have to. A long practice can be lazy and indulgent because we don't discipline the mind as much – we let it wander here there and everywhere as we go through our practice half-heartedly.

So don't get hung up on time. Devote yourself to as little as seven minutes a day (and watch yourself naturally do longer).

Focus instead on depth of being – being present, being whole-hearted and disciplining the mind.

Process versus Outcome

Even in our yoga practice we can often get stuck on the goal we want to achieve – on getting to some place in the future that will never arrive – and so we lose the treasure of being in the process.

This desire to achieve a goal can get in the way of us practicing yoga. We want our yoga practice to give us something – we want results!

We want to be more flexible, we want to lose weight, we want peace, we want calm, we want want want! This wanting means we're focused on turning our yoga practice into *the thing that will give us* what we want. We're trying to make it *be* something in order to *get* something. In doing so, we miss out on enjoying our practice for what it is, and letting the results take care of themselves.

The whole point of Yoga is to step out of doing and into being. Yoga is process. When we're practicing yoga, we're practicing being present. We open to and accept all that is arising in the moment. We stay with all the feelings and sensations arising in our bodies. We observe our mind, knowing we're not our thoughts.

That's all process. It's got nothing to do with achievements like touching our toes. You can't achieve yoga. Yoga is an allowing. You allow your mind to still. You allow your heart to open. You allow your awareness to settle on your breath. You allow your breath to fill your entire body. You allow yourself to drop into the present.

This shift from yoga as something we *do*, to yoga as something we *are*, is crucial if you want to maintain a life-long yoga practice.

Letting go of outcome and focusing on process also means you broaden your understanding of yoga as something that happens on the yoga mat and something that *also* happens *off* the yoga mat.

We go to our mat to practice this state of being called yoga. We also begin to take it off the mat with us. On the days when we never get to the mat, we can consciously work at dropping into this state of being no matter what it is we're doing.

We can be Yoga while parenting, while cleaning, while working, while exercising. There's no results to be achieved in any of this, no boxes to tick, no sense of accomplishment because we did ninety minutes of asana. But there is a process at work, subtly changing our perception and understanding of the world until the illusions drop and we see what is.

That's Yoga. Seeing what is. Being with what is.

Focusing on process over results means we allow ourselves the time to be in Yoga every single day. At first, maybe for years or decades, that means we get on our mats.

In time, being on the mat bleeds off the mat and we see that we've taken the practice of yoga into every part of our life. This is what happens when we focus on process instead of outcome.

Learn to enjoy the process, the outcome takes care of itself.

Conclusion

Our ideas of what a home yoga practice is can get in the way of us even having a practice. Broadening and deepening our definition of a home yoga practice helps to blast through these ideas and change the way we perceive our practice.

Yoga is not asana, it is not pranayama or chanting, or even meditation. Yoga is a path, a process and a destination. That destination is ultimately a state of being where we identify with our deeper Self, rather than the personality, or ego/mind.

When we create a home yoga practice, we're using tools and techniques to help us access and practice that state of being.

Going to class is an important way to learn some of the tools and techniques. However, Yoga is a personal practice that will differ for every individual person, based on their needs.

When we practice at home, we honour our individual Selves and needs. We also teach ourselves how to connect, listen to and trust our inner guidance.

Our home yoga practice will evolve as we evolve. There are four stages:
  - The need for specific postures and practices to support the learning.
  - The ability to vary postures and practices based on moon cycles, seasons and balancing the body, mind and emotions.
  - Heightened sensitivity leading to an awareness of what kind of practice is needed to support the body, mind or emotions.
  - A deep awareness of Prana, and the ability to surrender to its flow and allow it to guide the practice.

Movement through these stages will often correspond to a shift from a predominantly asana-based practice to a mostly-meditative practice.

Committing to forty continuous days gives us an easily achievable goal whilst re-wiring the psyche. Allowing ourselves to only practice seven minutes a day gets us on the mat no matter what: this may serve to deepen our practice because we value the time more intensely.

Watching our mind-state around our practice – something to do, achieve, succeed at, control, or dominate versus being, allowing, flowing, surrendering to – helps us to shift our relationship to yoga, and to the practice. Shifting this relationship to yoga and our practice helps yoga to become part of our lives, instead of just something we do on the mat.

Our ideal home yoga practice can be as little as seven minutes a day spent doing a personalised practice of asana, pranayama, chanting and/or meditation. It's a practice that teaches us how to drop into the state of being that is Yoga.

Simply put, a home yoga practice gives us time to practice Being.

That's it. Time to practice Being.

Time to Be.

Time.

To

Be.

What Stops You From Practicing?

It doesn't matter who we are – a newbie to home yoga practice, an experienced home practitioner or even a yoga teacher – our home yoga practice is a work in progress.

As our lives shift and change, so too do the reasons we practice or don't practice. Part of creating a practice and sticking to it is being able to identify all the obstacles that might come up. So when one does, we can immediately take action to deal with it whilst remaining focused on doing our home practice.

In reality, this means if we're about to have a baby, or start a new job with different hours, or move to a new country, *before* the change happens, we assess how it's going to impact our practice, and how our practice might need to shift and change.

When we don't do this work and expect our practice to stay the same even though our life is changing, we get caught out. Our practice fades away or drops completely and we struggle to bring it back. Staying ahead of the game means we can make the necessary changes to our practice as our lives change, making the transitions smooth, supportive and realistic.

Let's look at some of the common obstacles to a home yoga practice, the ways we can acknowledge the reality of these obstacles and identify strategies to deal with them.

Time

The number one reason people don't practice yoga at home is because they don't have enough time.

This is not true.

The number one reason people don't practice yoga at home is because *they perceive or believe* that they don't have enough time.

This is true.

What's the difference?

Perception and belief.

You have enough time to practice yoga:

- if you make it a priority in your day
- if you take time to figure out where it best fits in
- if you let go of the idea a home yoga practice needs to be at least an hour long to make it worthwhile.

We've already talked about the seven minute practice. You know you can fit that into your life, and any extra time after seven minutes is a bonus.

So, the first step in making time for a home yoga practice is examining your beliefs and perception of time: then making up your mind that you do have enough time to practice.

You have enough time to practice yoga.

Now find it. Even if it is just seven minutes. (Found it yet?)

Don't think that your time, however long it is, has to be at the same time every day.

Consistency and regularity makes a habit easier to stick with, so in an ideal world you would practice at the same time every single day.

But you don't have to.

You can practice whenever you like, whenever you need to, whenever you can fit it in.

Once upon a time, I had a city job involving a forty minute bus ride each way. I practiced yoga on the bus every morning and every afternoon. No, I wasn't doing Downward Dogs in the aisle or Twists in my seat. I was chanting. Silently. I kept my feet grounded, my spine erect, my awareness on my breath, and I repeated my mantra over and over and over again. I even had my hands folded in my lap in a mudra.

By the time my bus arrived and I disembarked, I felt clear, calm, grounded and ready to start my working day. As I walked the remaining ten minutes to work, I switched from a mantra to a walking meditation. My awareness was still on my breath, but also on my feet on the ground and my spine extending towards the sky.

At work, during lunch hour I would take my yoga mat outside on fine days to a close-by patch of lawn and do a thirty-minute asana practice, before eating lunch and heading back to the office.

Put all this together, and I was edging towards two hours of dedicated yoga practice, while working a full time job with a lengthy commute.

You can do the same in your life. If you want to. So take some time now to look over your diary or calendar and identify when you could practice yoga in your day, and in your week.

–   What does your average day and your average week look like?
–   What time do you get out of bed?
–   When do you have down time?
–   What activities currently fill up your day that are less important to you than yoga?
–   Could you skip a TV program you watch regularly?
–   Would you get up earlier to practice yoga?
–   Can you practice in your lunch break?

Your focus here is not on seeing the lack of time, the difficulties or the issues. You're looking for solutions, work-arounds and good-enoughs.

Look hard, make some priority calls, shift some things around and you'll soon see that if you want to make time for a yoga practice, you can. Every. Single. Day.

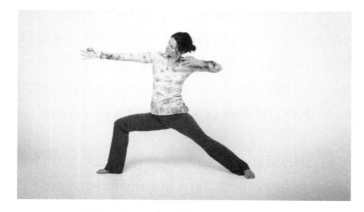

Take aim – find time to practice

Worksheet 1: Time

Action 1:
In Column One write all the possible times you could practice yoga.

Action 2:
In Column Two write the changes you would need to make in your life.

Possible Times I could Practice (be creative)	Change I need to make first
In the morning	Get up twenty minutes earlier
At the sports fields while my son practices soccer	Getting over being seen in public practicing yoga
After work	Leave earlier to miss traffic

Place

After time, the biggest reason people have for not practicing yoga is they don't have the perfect place.

This is true.

Many people *don't* have the perfect place for practicing – they may have small bedrooms, small houses, flatmates, family members, a busy house, no yoga mat.

In an ideal world, you would have a permanent spot for your yoga mat dedicated just to yoga and meditation. The lighting would be soft, there would be a beautiful view and it would be cozy and warm.

But here's the thing.

You don't *need* any of this to practice yoga. You don't even need a yoga mat. All you need is a single-pointed desire to find the best place for your yoga practice that you can.

Let's take a look. Check out your house. Check out your bedroom. Check out other spaces you have available to you in your regular life – like your workplace or place of study. Get creative – do you have a friend who also wants to develop a regular home yoga practice and has space you could use?

There's always somewhere to practice.

In the worst case scenario, the limitations of space will place limitations on your yoga practice, but it doesn't mean you can't still practice. You can practice yoga sitting on a long-haul flight in coach. Maybe it would be mostly pranayama, mudra, silent chanting and meditation with the odd twist or forward-bend but it's still yoga.

So what's your best case scenario based on your space? Is there somewhere you could dedicate to yoga?

No dedicated space? Then here are some good spaces to practice:

In the kitchen.

Most kitchens are big enough for a yoga mat, the floor is usually firm but not too hard. There's the added bonus of benches which make great support and props. Kitchens have less traffic than lounges and it's ok to make the kitchen off-limits at certain times of the day. Like after 8pm.

In the lounge.

The floor can be soft, there's usually plenty of space for a mat. Sometimes there's even a nice view or a fire to focus on. Claim the lounge for a set amount of time every day.

Hallways.

Great space for yoga because you have the walls for support and they are usually clear of any kind of clutter. It's also easy to put up some kind of wall hanging to make the space more yoga-like. Whatever that means to you.

Porches, balconys, backyards, garages, gazebos and sheds.

Don't get stuck inside the house. If you live in a place where the weather is settled most of the year, get outside and soak up the elements.

I have a friend who practices under a large oak tree whenever the weather permits, and he swears by it, often finishing his practice with meditation up the tree. Outside – and spaces open to the outside – offer their own challenges and their own rewards.

Workspaces.

There is nowhere better in a busy work life than practicing at work. Yes, you have to get over the worry about what people will think of you, or if people will watch you. Likely though, you'll inspire people. Think meeting rooms, spare rooms, beside your desk, in your office, in a co-worker's office, in the storage room, in the server room, in the kitchen. Wherever.

Don't forget about outside your work either. I used to practice on the back lawns of Parliament, beside my office block. Beautiful spot in the sun! Later, an MP's secretary happened to mention the woman who practiced yoga on Parliament's lawns and how inspiring it was... he had no idea it was me.

You never know who you might impact when you're brave enough to take your practice out into the big wide world. Imagine a world where people practicing yoga in public was as common as people eating junk food on the street.

I have another friend who drives into work early so he can do his morning practice in his workspace before anybody else arrives. By the time they rock in, he's done a sixty-minute practice or so, and just has to change into his work clothes. It's also making his work colleagues interested in yoga.

Ok, I know, some of these suggestions may freak you out – practice beside my desk, are you crazy! Outside in public? Mad! But you know what, do you want to practice daily or not?

Well? Do you want to do this?

Then make it happen. Work with what you've got, get over yourself and make it happen. Outside isn't so bad. Beside your desk, early, when the office is mostly empty, isn't so bad. Bring a friend if you can. There's always safety in numbers.

Finally, if you travel a lot, think about where you go. Flying? Airports? Hotels? Friends' houses? Where can you practice along the way?

Some airports actually have dedicated yoga spaces now, and it's not hard to find a quiet spot in an airport to set up a mat and do a discreet seated posture sequence. It's all about working with what you have.

In our non-ideal world, practicing in the same space most of the time works best. There's something about the resonance that builds up when we do the same activity over and over and over again in that space. But it doesn't matter if it's the kitchen, the workplace or the local park.

All that matters is you make the best of what's available to you, and have several possible spaces for practice lined up for the times when someone's cooking, watching TV, or having a hall party.

Variety will make it more likely that you'll stick to your practice.

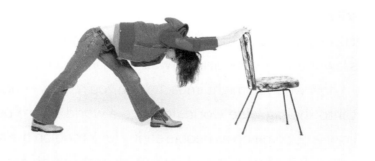

Any place can be a practice place.

Worksheet 2: Places and Spaces to Practice Yoga

> **Action 1:**
> Write all the places you regularly spend time.

> **Action 2:**
> Write all the spaces for each place where you could practice.

Places I spend time	Spaces I could practice
Home	Lounge in the the morning Bedroom at night Lawn on a nice sunny day
Work	Meeting room Grassy park across the street
Traveling	In my hotel room In the hotel gym.

What to do?

After time and place, the next biggest reason people don't practice yoga at home is because they don't know what to do. Nobody likes feeling like they don't know, it's uncomfortable. Well, get used to it. Yoga is about getting out of our comfort zone and moving into the unknown. It's ok not to know. It's *great* not to know!

And there are ways to find out. The question is then, how do you find out?

First step, *resolve* to work it out. Decide that you will figure out what it is you need to practice at home. Decide that you are capable of working out – with the help of resources and other people – what it is you're going to do in your home yoga practice.

Here are some ways you can figure out what to do in your home yoga practice:
- Find a book that outlines a practice you want to follow
- Do a one-on-one session with a teacher who sets you a home practice
- Design your own home practice session based on the information we gather through later worksheets
- Practice along with a DVD until you learn the sequence
- Sign up for an on-line yoga course that teaches you a set sequence
- Set acceptable parameters for your level of experience and work within those. E.g. I'll do ten minutes of standing postures, ten minutes of sitting postures and a closing sequence of a backbend, a twist and Corpse Pose
- Find a specific Kriya and learn that practice

There is *always* a way to figure out what to do. The point is you start where you are, with what you know. Then seek out available resources to expand your knowledge, incorporating it into your home practice over time.

My home practice started when I came home from overseas and was living back at home, in a tiny town in the middle of nowhere with not a hint of a yoga class nearby. I don't think I even had the Internet.

I had a choice. Don't practice, or do what I could.

In the four years previous, I'd done some Ashtanga yoga and some Bikram yoga. It was just enough to give me an idea of the outline of a practice – standing, seated, closing. Based on that and generally starting with sun salutations, I did yoga of some sort most days. Sure, it wasn't fantastic. I may have put postures together that didn't quite belong together. But I was practicing and felt better after I'd practiced than before.

Later, I bought Beryl Bender Birch's book *Power Yoga* and used that as my home sequence. I moved onto a Baron Baptiste DVD and learned that. Bit by bit, over time and with persistence and dedication, I learned more and more yoga while developing a home practice that has stuck with me to this day.

You too can do that.

Later, we'll look at why you want to do a home yoga practice and the answer to that question will help guide you towards creating your perfect home yoga practice. But for now ask yourself:

'What is it you know right now about yoga?'

'If you were to stop reading this book right now and do some yoga, what could you do?'

That's enough. That's a starting point, and that is all you need. Somewhere to start.

Worksheet 3: Possible Yoga Practices

> **Action 1:**
> **What do you know about yoga right now?**

What I know about Yoga
Child's Pose, Corpse Pose, Mountain Pose
Sun Salutation
Deep belly breathing

Naysayers and Distracters

People, people, people everywhere.

We live with people. We work with people. We hang out with people. We go out with people.

Not all of these people are going to be supportive, understanding and encouraging of your yoga practice.

While most won't be naysayers, many will be distracters. Children for one – great distracters! Partners – who wouldn't rather curl up on the couch with a loved one rather than hit the yoga mat?

Getting clear on the role that the people in your life play in your home yoga practice is a key element to knowing how to work around them. Take some time now to think about all the people in your life – those you live with and work with, those you love and those you hang out with.

Of those people, who is likely to distract you from your practice the most and in what way?

Of those people, who are likely to talk negatively (even in a joking way) about your practice and about you doing your practice?

Now, how are you going to deal with those people?

- Can you bring them onside?
- Can you neutralise them?
- Can you kick them out of your life? (I mean seriously – someone doesn't want you to practice yoga? What's with that?)

I know. You probably can't kick them out of your life. Not if it's a child who'll want your attention, a mate who gets sulky, a mother-in-law who's sniffy about yoga or a boss who thinks it's all woo-woo. But you can work with them... you can always work with them.

Here's what to ask yourself about the Naysayers:

- Do I have to tell them I'm practicing yoga every day?

- Can I have a heart-to-heart with them prior to starting my Forty Days of Yoga and get them onside?
- Am I strong enough to assert my boundary – i.e. tell them this is important for me and I'm going to do my practice even if they attempt to sidetrack me?
- If I'm not strong enough to assert a boundary (and that's something to work on), what else could I do?

Is there a trusted friend who could help me brainstorm up a tactic?

Don't be tempted to skip this section. Don't think, oh it's ok, everyone's fine. It's really, *really* important that you look at all the people you interact with regularly and ascertain whether or not they're going to support you.

Otherwise, it will be Friday night at 7pm and you won't have practiced and your best friend will drop by with a bottle of wine and… what's going to happen?

- If she's a supporter and you're wavering about practice, she'll tell you to go and do your twenty minutes right now while she pours the wine and plates the cheeses. She'll hold the line for you. Yoga first, then wine.
- If she's a distracter and you waver, she won't hold the line for you. It'll be wine o'clock.
- If she's a naysayer, she'll laugh and tell you about the relaxing properties of wine. Why waste time on the mat when you could be drinking?

We all have days when we waver – that's when we turn to our supporters (more on them later). Those are the days we avoid the naysayers and the distracters.

Worksheet 4: Naysayers and Distracters

Action 1:
Look at the people in your life.
Are they a naysayer or a distractor?

Action 2:
Write at least one strategy per person to minimize the effect
they have on you and your life. Add them to the correct column.

Naysayers	Distracters	Strategies
Boss – Hates Yoga		Don't talk about yoga around the boss; don't ask to do it in any workspace.
	Best Friend – loves to party.	Have a heart to heart with her and explain why this is important.

Procrastination

There's always something else we could be doing, and there's often something else we'd rather be doing than our home yoga practice.

I'll do it after breakfast, I'll do it after lunch, I'll do it after work, I'll do it after dinner. I'll do it after this TV show. I'll do it before bed. I'll do it… tomorrow.

Ah yes, procrastination. It's a golden rule of life that if we took all the energy we use to procrastinate about doing something and instead applied it to doing the thing… it would have been done yesterday already. Or last week. Or last month.

You will procrastinate.

There will be something better to do.

But procrastination is never just putting something off. There's always a reason *why* we want to put that something off. Procrastination is 'I don't want to because…'

But you want to, right? You want a home yoga practice?

So procrastination may have stopped you in the past, but it's not going to stop you this time.

Procrastination is just an excuse and you'll learn how to deal with it later. Once you actually start your practice. Worrying about procrastination *now* is a form of procrastination itself. So let's just get on with it.

Perfectionism versus Good Enough

> *'I'll start a home practice when I have a ninety minute chunk of time available every day.'*
> *'I'll start a home practice when I have a dedicated yoga room.'*
> *'I'll start a home yoga practice when I know the entire Ashtanga sequence off by heart.'*
> *'I'll start when my kids start going to school.'*
> *'I'll start when the kids move out.'*
> *'I'll start when I lose some weight.'*
> *'I'll start when…'*

There will never be a more perfect time to start your home yoga practice than today. Now is the perfect time.

As we've clearly seen in the previous pages, you don't need a whole lot of time, you don't need a whole lot of space, you don't need to know exactly what you're doing and you don't need to wait until you're surrounded by supportive people.

Perfectionism is just procrastination, dressed up in better clothing. It's another way of holding on, another way of resisting, another way of attempting to control life.

You don't need it.

All you need is good enough.

Good enough gets you on your mat or carpet or tiles or towel or sand or grass. Good enough sees you practicing for seven or fifteen or sixty-three minutes. Good enough is sun salutations only. Yoga Nidra at night. Chanting silently on the bus. Good enough is faded track pants and baggy t-shirts. Good enough is muting the ads and putting in five minutes before your favourite TV show comes back on. That's good enough. (We have long ad-breaks in New Zealand – long enough to practice yoga in!)

Good enough gets you going and once you get going, you're opening up to possibility.

Opening up to possibility means when you get on your mat for ten minutes because that's all you think you have... then there's a possibility you'll stay twenty minutes because it feels so good.

Opening up to possibility means you practice in your kitchen every single morning, and make sure the next house you rent has a dedicated yoga space.

Opening up to possibility means those five sun salutations become deeper and more present until you easily do forty sun salutations and enjoy every single moment of it.

That's where good enough takes you. Into a field of possibility and that field is what will support your home yoga practice.

Guilt

When most people think about why they don't practice this is not an obvious answer.

Guilt? About what?

About enjoying oneself too much. About indulging in time out. About taking time out from the family and from work obligations. About doing something just for ourselves.

That's what.

I notice it's a strong reason why I don't practice especially when my son is in childcare and therefore I have time. This is also the time I devote to my business and I feel guilty about stopping to practice yoga. I'm my own boss! I could stop and practice for two hours and no one would get upset at me. But I don't. There's a voice inside saying:

'You should be working. You should be making money. You should be productive.'

This voice is insidious. Mostly because society constantly validates it. Working hard and pushing yourself beyond your own limits is seen as some kind of heroic act. Taking time out and looking after yourself at the perceived expense of work can be seen as indulgent and lazy.

Guilt can be a strong emotion for parents. We're already doing so much, usually balancing running a house with work and bringing up children. Something is always demanding our attention. Finding time to practice yoga amongst all of those demands just doesn't seem important. We put our kids first. We put our work first. We put looking after the house first. We put our community first, our friends first, our family first.

Even for those of us without kids, there are still all those other demands and it can be difficult to acknowledge that we matter too.

Regardless, our practice makes us better people. It makes us more able to withstand the demands of modern life and all that tugs at us. We become better parents, better work colleagues, better bosses, better friends and better family members.

Realising that guilt is what stops us from practicing is a powerful step forward. Guilt is based on an idea that everything else is more important than our own well-being, and that's not true. Once we see that guilt holds us back we can address it head on. Which we'll do after we look at one last obstacle to practicing yoga daily. Or nine of them.

Patanjali's Obstacles

There are other more devious obstacles that will arise when you commit to your *Forty Days of Yoga*. Fortunately for us, these obstacles are known foes and have been famous amongst yogis for centuries.

In fact, this is one of the most awesome things about traveling the path of yoga – knowing that while you have to do it by yourself and experience it for yourself, other people have walked this path before and experienced exactly the same things as you. Just in different ways.

These pioneers of the path, like Patanjali (although he's not the only person who has written about yoga and its path), reassure us that whatever we're facing is natural, normal and just part of the ride.

(Patanjali was an early yogi and scholar who compiled and wrote yoga wisdom into a collection of sutras, or threads, known simply as Yoga Sutras).

So take heart, don't get distracted: stay with your practice. Patanjali has been there, done that, and has written the roadmap to help you through.

So what does Patanjali have to say about obstacles?

Briefly, there's nine of them. They give rise to four more. Without the first nine, you don't get the next four. But you're most likely to spot the four in yourself first, because they're more obvious. When you spot one of the four, you can be sure that beneath the surface lurks one of the nine. The nine are more subtle.

The four are grosser.

Nine Predictable Obstacles to a Home Yoga Practice:
- Vyadhi = disease, illness, sickness
- Styana = mental laziness, inefficiency, idleness, procrastination, dullness

- Samshaya = indecision, doubt
- Pramada = carelessness, negligence
- Alasya = sloth, languor, laziness
- Avirati = sensuality, want of non-attachment, non-abstention, craving
- Bhranti-darshana = false views or perception, confusion of philosophies
- Alabdha-bhumikatva = failing to attain stages of practice
- Anavasthitatva = instability, slipping down, inability to maintain

Their Four Lovely Companions:
- Duhkha = pain (mental or physical)
- Daurmanasya = sadness, despair, dejection, frustration, depression, anguish
- Angam-ejayatva = shakiness, unsteadiness, movement, tremor of the limbs or body
- Shvasa and preshvasah = (irregular)inhalation, inspiration and (irregular) exhalation, expiration

You can read all about these in Patanjali's Sutras, specifically Sutra 1.30 – 1.32. Find a good translation. Even better, buy a good translation. (Try Desikachar's *'Heart of Yoga'*, listed in the resources). On days when you hit an obstacle you can dip into the Sutras and be reminded that it's all par for the course.

The key element to remember here is that the Nine Obstacles begin as a distraction – which holds the potential of an obstacle – but a distraction hasn't yet become an obstacle. It's only shown up in our field of awareness. If we notice that we're experiencing Styana (such as procrastination) and choose to hold the line and stay focused on our practice regardless of the feeling of 'can't be bothered' we're experiencing... then Styana *hasn't* turned into an obstacle. Our focus has dealt with the distraction.

And that's what matters.

See the distraction. Know that every yogi encounters these distractions along the way. Don't let it distract you *and* become an obstacle.

What you do with it is what counts. What we're going to do with it is practice.

Oh, and if you get stuck doing this worksheet then it's time to phone a friend. Check in with someone else – a friend, a yoga teacher, a family member – and ask them how they would deal with the issues that you're uncovering.

At the end of this exercise you will have multiple ways to deal with all the reasons why you don't practice yoga. This is possibility and potential. This is you taking charge of your home yoga practice and seeing all the choices you have around creating this practice.

What you will realise as you go through this experience, is that there is *one thing and one thing only that will keep you practicing yoga* every single day.

Your unwavering desire to do so.

Patanjali calls it one-pointedness. I like to call it bloody-mindedness.

I. Will. Practice. And so will you. Every day.

Worksheet 5: What Stops You From Practicing?

> **Action 1:**
> **Answer this question.**
> **Why don't you practice yoga at home every day?**

Write at least twenty responses to this question, using a full statement every time. If you start to run out of obstacles, make 'em silly. Make 'em ridiculous. Make 'em up. Get those twenty responses down.

The reasons I don't practice yoga
I don't have enough time in my day.
I don't have a dedicated yoga space.
I'm too tired after I put my child to bed.
I feel guilty about taking time out
All I want to do is have a glass of wine while I'm cooking and I can't practice after that.
Work is more important than practicing.
Asana makes me feel dizzy and my body is not up for it.
I can't be bothered.
I don't think it matters anymore.

Action 2:
Read each statement out loud and ask yourself, 'Is this true?'
Write True or Untrue in Column 1.

True?	Reasons For Not Practicing
No	I don't have enough time in my day.
Yes	I don't have a dedicated yoga space.
Yes	I'm too tired after I put my son to bed.
Yes	I feel guilty about taking time out
Yes	All I want to do is have a glass of wine while I'm cooking and I can't practice after that.
No	Work is more important than practicing.
Sometimes	Asana makes me feel dizzy and my body is not up for it.
Sometimes	I can't be bothered.
No	I don't think it matters anymore.

Firstly, let's deal with the statements that aren't true.

If they aren't true then why are they stopping you from practicing yoga?

Because they're an excuse, that's why. So let's answer them. If for example you wrote: 'I don't have enough time in my day.'

You're going to answer with the time you do have, or could make available.

'I could get up ten minutes earlier each day and practice.' 'I could practice as soon as my son goes to childcare for twenty minutes.'

'I could practice for thirty minutes as soon as my son goes to bed at 7pm.'

Action 3:
Go through all of the untrue statements and write as many answers and as many possibilities as you can.

Untrue Statements	Workarounds
I don't have time in in my day.	I just did the Time Worksheet and discovered I have all the time I can use
Work is more important than practicing.	Who says? Practicing yoga makes my work go so much better. I can concentrate better after practice.

Now let's attend to the statements you wrote that are stopping you from practicing yoga, and that *are* true.

> **Action 4:**
> **Go through all the statements and find work-arounds for them.**

True Statements	Workarounds
I'm too tired after I put my son to bed.	I could do a restorative practice. I could meditate. I could do pranayama. I could do yoga nidra. I could find time earlier in my day.
Work is more important than practicing.	Who says? Practicing yoga makes my work go so much better. I can concentrate better after practice.

Excellent! Now there are no reasons left why you can't practice yoga every day. You're on your way!

The Benefits of Yoga

Do enough research and it seems we can find evidence that regular practice of yoga can positively impact everything from anxiety, depression, panic attacks, thyroid conditions, sciatica and asthma. It could be said that yoga can positively impact anything that has to do with the functioning of our physical bodies, minds or emotions.

How can this be possible? Surely yoga is not a silver bullet?

Well no, it's not.

However, yoga works to harmonise the body, mind and emotions by removing blockages at all levels of our system. The removal of these blockages allow our bodies, minds and emotions to function at their optimum level.

Yoga is often referred to as the Science of Life, and with good reason. Over the centuries yogis have used the practice of yoga (in its broadest dimensions) to experientially collect information about the way we function. This information has been codified for easy explanation and now the work of Western scientists is corroborating more and more of what the yogis learned experientially (and of what you will experience as you go deeper and deeper into your practice).

However, this is not the place to go in-depth into yoga worldview, or the myriad of positive impacts yoga can have on you. We've got *Forty Days of Yoga* to get stuck into.

Right now, just remember that yoga has both tangible and intangible benefits. Mostly, we start practicing because of the tangible benefits – like thinner thighs, increased flexibility, happier relationships, improved self esteem and greater lung capacity.

Over time though, it's the intangible benefits that keep us coming back to our mat.

Our mind feels clearer and we're able to handle our emotions better. Life becomes more joyful and we feel more capable of handling whatever it throws at us.

Who wouldn't want that?

The Benefits of a Home Practice

Our entire life, we're trained to look outside of ourselves for everything we need – social cues on how to behave, approval, the right way to do things, pleasure, fun, good times. Whatever we need, we'll find it outside of ourselves, right?

Wrong.

This is one of the major benefits of a home yoga practice – we learn to rely on what's *inside* of ourselves for all our needs. Yes, *all* our needs. This is the evolution of Self.

Yes, we still need food, water and shelter to keep our body functioning. But beyond that we become self-contained and able to meet our own needs. We can recognise our needs and we can take the action required to meet them.

Practicing yoga at home by ourselves means we're willing to take responsibility for ourselves and look after our own needs. It means we're shifting from being a passive receiver or victim of life, to an empowered chooser and responder to life.

You don't get that in class. Or rather, when you start to tune into that aspect of Self in class, you may find it more and more difficult to go to class because you'll start noticing when a class isn't what you need right now. You'll get in a terrible bind as you attempt to honour the teacher at the front of the room while still honouring the teacher within.

The blessings of cultivating your own inner wisdom and the ability to tune into your own needs and meet them spills over into every other aspect of your life. You'll know not to trust that guy who seems like the perfect date. You'll know to trust saying "yes" to that job even though it means taking a pay cut.

Going to class isn't bad, having a teacher isn't bad. Going to class can be crucial to give us a sense of community. It also helps us learn new ways of approaching yoga and ensures we're not blind to our own Selves. I'd recommend that you continue to work with a teacher in whatever capacity is available to you.

But the evolution of Self – which is really what this yoga path is all about – requires that at some point, we take charge of our own lives.

And your home yoga practice?

That's you taking charge.

You're becoming master of your Self.

The Benefits of a Yoga Toolbox

Sometimes life sucks and it throws us giant curve balls. At these times, it pays to have some great deal-to-life tools in the toolbox. I don't mean a bottle of wine or a six pack of beer. Sure, those distractions may momentarily dull your pain, but afterwards they'll leave you feeling worse than ever.

Not so yoga.

Over time and with practice you can build up a set of Yogic Tools to meet any life challenge.

When you're faced with a life challenge that you don't yet have a Yogic Tool for, you'll have the resources and connections to find the right tool.

Here are some examples of using Yogic Tools to cope with life challenges:

- New born baby, broken sleep, serious exhaustion? Try using Yoga Nidra recordings. Every time your baby goes to sleep, make yourself take a nap and start with a thirty minute Yoga Nidra. Worth two hours deep sleep at least.
- Back issues? Gentle back-specific asana with visualization.
- Emotional disturbance? Ten sun salutations with a strong focus on Ujjiya breath.
- Anxiety? Meditation with appropriate mantra.
- Muddled mind and can't figure out what to do? Alternate Nostril Breathing.
- Exhausted and recovering from illness? Try twenty minutes of restorative yoga.

No matter what challenge you're facing, you will always feel better after some yoga.

When you practice at home on a regular basis, you're honing your ability to tune in and see what it is that you need.

Plus you get a chance to practice various tools, whether it's strong asana, gentle asana, pranayama, meditation, yoga nidra, chanting or visualisation. When you need that tool, you know it inside-out. It's second nature for you to practice it.

Two years after coming back to New Zealand, my yoga practice was helping me process emotion, but I still felt anxious, ungrounded, and had muddled thinking.

A day-long workshop with Swami Shantimurti of Ashram Yoga proved a huge turning point in my recovery from psychosis.

First he was able to validate my intuition that my mental break with reality had a spiritual component and second, he was able to give me specific practices to help me work through the blockages in my mind and emotions.

Huge relief.

Finally, a yogic tool specifically designed to help me.

What a difference it made in my life.

I still practice Alternate Nostril Breathing on a regular basis today. It calms my mind, grounds me and helps me to find clarity. Plus, it also balances the left and right hemispheres of the brain, helping to clear out the two major nadis, Pingala and Ida.

It was just what I needed.

Your home yoga practice will be able to do that for you too.

Imagine sitting in a hospital, caring for a loved one. It's so easy to get sucked into fear and worry and anxiety. But when you know yoga, you know you can hold your bedside vigil while repeating a loving-kindness meditation. You know you've got choices.

That's the power of a home yoga practice. That's the power of having a Yogic Toolbox. It's not something you can ever buy but, boy oh boy, are you grateful for taking the time to build it when the time arises for it.

A yogi toolbox is something that builds over time, but right now it's likely you already have some challenging situations in your life where yoga could help.

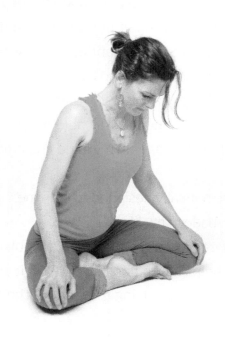

Sitting still with awareness helps us shift state

Worksheet 6: Building a Yogic Toolbox

> **Action 1:**
> **In Column One write a list of the**
> **challenging situations in your life.**

> **Action 2:**
> **In Column Two write out any**
> **yogic solutions you already know about.**

Challenging Situation	Possible Yogic Solutions
Chronic back issues	Gentle asana that focus on releasing the hip flexors, including legs up the wall, lunges.

It doesn't matter if you don't know any yoga solutions – this is just a starting point. Later, you can research and find specific solutions for challenges you face.

This list is something that will grow and expand over time – keep it close and add to it frequently.

Harnessing Your Motivation

Wanting a home yoga practice can be a bit like wanting to write a book. Often, what we really want are the results of the experience, not the experience itself.

Someone might want to be interviewed, make a swag of money, end up on Oprah, and have millions of people reading their work. They don't actually want to sit at the computer day after day and write, sweating blood and tears until they've produced something great.

It can be the same with a home yoga practice.

Sometimes we can really want to be thin, flexible, calm, and peaceful. But when it comes to getting on the mat every day and actually being with the sometimes horrible experience of those ninety (or seven) minutes: *that* part we don't want.

Our focus is on wanting the outcome, not experiencing the process. Yoga, like life, is all process. Outcomes are incidental.

It's time to be honest with yourself.

Are you motivated to practice because you want to experience the results or is it because you want the experience of practicing yoga every day?

Either answer is ok – there is no right or wrong. Honesty is crucial so we can respond to our true motivation.

Yoga is about making the unconscious conscious, so this is our Yoga, right here right now, figuring out what's driving us – really driving us to practice yoga at home.

Ironically, deep suffering can be the best possible motivation for a home yoga practice, because we're so desperate to make a change in our lives and feel better.

My shift from yoga classes to a home practice came at the absolute worst time of my life.

It was October 2004 and at the age of twenty-nine I was back living in New Zealand, at my Mum's house. In the months previous, I'd had two psychotic episodes and been committed to an acute psych ward in Vancouver, my fiance had broken up with me, and my financial situation had completely collapsed.

I was a wreck – broken-minded, broken-hearted and just plain broke.

Even in the psych ward in Canada, I knew that yoga was going to save me. It had to – nothing else could.

On the days when the weather allowed us outside of the psych unit onto the grassed lawn, I'd go through a few sun salutations, albeit half-heartedly. It was the only thing I knew that could give me some relief from my crazed mind.

Even then, my preference was to go to class and be told what to do, to have a teacher who cared about me take me under their wing and look after me. To have someone else be responsible for my needs.

It wasn't to be though. I spent nine days in that psych ward, before being released, and with no choice but to leave the life I'd spent seven years building in Whistler, and head home to New Zealand.

In my overseas absence, my mother had taken a job as the principal of a small school in rural Glenorchy (population 400 odd), so that was where I ended up.

There was no yoga. All I could do was unroll a mat on the concrete pad that served as a deck at the schoolhouse my Mum was renting and do what I could remember.

Later, when I moved to Queenstown – a thriving resort town in the heart of New Zealand's South Island – I did go to a few classes and I despaired. My consciousness-expanding experiences hadn't just lead to psychosis: they'd also taken me way past the idea of yoga as exercise, and the teachers I encountered seemed to still regard yoga as something one did with one's body.

Nothing wrong with that: it is one step on the yoga journey. But it wasn't where I was, nor was it what I needed or wanted as my practice.

Classes didn't deliver what I needed to help me deal with my broken heart and mind, so I had to turn inwards and find something within me to do it. I needed a home yoga practice.

It was a huge motivation for beginning a home yoga practice and it worked. Desperation can bring us to the mat, day in and day out because we know that life can be better than this. That we are better than this.

Your reasons for wanting a home practice could be something much less desperate and range from anything like losing weight, gaining flexibility, cultivating calmness or exploring yoga deeper.

It might be that, like me, you have no choice because you don't live close to classes.

Whatever it is, the reasons why you want a home yoga practice will inform both what you do in your practice and how likely you are to stick to that practice.

Over time too, the reasons why you want a home yoga practice will shift and change. My desperate need for equanimity has faded, as it has become an ingrained part of my life. In some ways, losing this desperation has made it more difficult to stick to my home practice, because I don't need it so badly. Being conscious of this change of motivation means I have to motivate myself in other ways.

More on that later. First, what is motivating your home yoga practice?

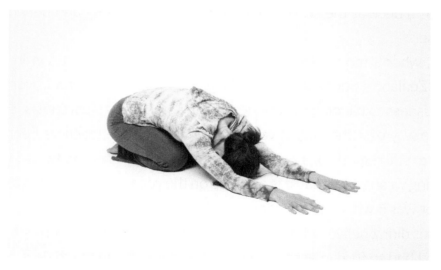

Child's Pose is sometimes called the Wisdom Pose because it helps us rest deep inside ourselves.

Worksheet 7: Assessing Your Yoga Needs

Getting clear on why you need to practice yoga is a powerful process. So is knowing the benefits of a yoga practice, and specifically a home yoga practice. Knowing what your needs are – physical, mental, emotional and spiritual – will help you figure out what to do in your practice.

> **Action 1:**
> **Write down all the physical reasons you need to practice yoga.**

The physical reasons I need to practice yoga
I want to be able to touch my toes
I want to improve the movement of my spine
I want to be able to do up my shoe laces
I want to be able to move my neck freely

Write and write and write until you can write no more.

Action 2:
Write all the mental reasons you want to practice yoga.

The mental reasons I need to practice yoga.
I want to have a clear and calm mind.
I want to alleviate my anxiety.
I want to shift my depression.

Action 3:
Write the emotional reason why you want to practice yoga.

The emotional reasons I need to practice yoga.
I want to have better relationships with my family.
I want to love myself more.
I want to release all the suppressed emotion from my childhood.

Action 4:
Write out your spiritual reasons for practicing yoga.

The spiritual reasons I need to practice yoga.
I want to know God.
I want to experience Oneness.
I don't believe in spirituality.

Whatever, it doesn't matter. The point of this exercise is just to get it all out as if you don't care what anybody thinks, least of all yourself, because you don't. Dig deep, be honest, get silly and write it all down.

Now. Take a break. Go do some yoga. Meditation. Pranayama. Turn some music on. Boogie in the lounge, whatever. Just get out of your head.

Once you've done that, come back and read everything that you're written down – all the reasons why you want to practice yoga. Take a different coloured pen, it doesn't matter. This is your process.

Action 5:
Read through the list and when you get to something important underline it, highlight it, put a star beside it.

Read fast and go with the first instinct. At the end you'll have something like five to ten really important reasons why you want to practice yoga.

Action 6:
Write a heading:
My Really Important Reasons for Practicing Yoga

Action 7:
Read through your underlined highlighted starred answers
and tick the ones that leap out at you.
There might be 3 or 4. Draw that many columns.

Action 8:
Write those underlined / highlighted / starred / ticked answers
under your heading, one item per column.

My Really Important Reasons for Practicing Yoga		
I want to love myself more.	I want to get to know God.	I want to be able to do up my own shoelaces.

These statements are why you want to have a home yoga practice and those reasons 'why' will guide what kind of home yoga practice you do.

In this instance, you may decide to start with Statement 3 and craft a practice that frees up the pelvis, spine and hamstrings so you can tie your shoelaces.

But we're going to take our diving into motivations down another level.

> **Action 9:**
> **Write those underlined / highlighted / starred / ticked answers under your heading, one item per column.**

Your Important Reason	Because – the reason why it's important
I want to love who I am...	because I want to love being myself.
I want to get to know God...	because everyone who's met him talks about him as if he's the dude to know.
I want to be able to tie my shoelaces up...	because I'm only 26 and I want to be independent and capable.

It doesn't matter what you write. There are no magic and correct answers here. There are only the answers that you make up. So if it feels like you're making them up, it's because you are!

You should now have a number of important reasons why you want to practice yoga, framed as '*Statement 1 because Answer 1*'.

Action 10:
Take each statement at the top of each column, and underneath
write out one sentence in the following format.
'When I *INSERT ANSWER 1* it will feel...

Important Reason	Because	I will feel
I want to love who I am.	I want to love being myself.	I will feel joyous and happy and able to cope with whatever life throws my way.
I want to get to know God.	Everyone who's met him talks about him as if he's the dude to know.	I will feel connected to something greater than myself.
I want to be able to tie my shoelaces easily.	I'm only 26 and I want to be independent and capable.	I will feel strong enough to cope with anything that comes my way.

These endings you've just written are the deeper reasons why you want to do a yoga practice. Not just for getting to the bottom of fear, not just to meet God and not just to tie up shoelaces... but to feel strong and capable, and at one with the Universe. You've now uncovered both your surface motivations and core motivations for wanting a home yoga practice.

The Principles of an Asana Practice

As you'll have realised by now, this book is not about how to do X, Y and Z postures so you have the perfect home practice. It's about the process around a home practice.

However, it does help to have some idea of *how* to practice asana, because most of you will be incorporating asana into your home yoga practice. These principles won't give you the *'What'* exactly, but they give you something to ground your asana practice in, so you have a sense that you know what you're doing.

You don't need to intimately know the correct anatomy and physiology of every yoga posture. All you need to know are the underlying principles of practicing asana. Knowing these underlying principles means you can turn any body position
– from sitting on your chair right now reading this book – into asana.

While the following principles apply mainly to the practice of asana, elements also hold true for other ways to practice yoga – like meditation or pranayama.

This is an overview designed to give you enough information to remember the principles, and to play with them in your home yoga practice. An entire book could be written about these alone!

Don't expect to take all these principles in, or know them all perfectly immediately. Developing an asana practice takes time, it shifts and grows as you learn. This gives you something to refer to and something to explore further in other reading.

Breath Connection

Without this principle you are not practicing yoga but merely doing gymnastics.

When you practice yoga you must be aware of your breath, because to be aware of your breath is to *be aware*. As you read these words right now, become aware of your inhale and your exhale. Listen to yourself breathe, feel yourself breathe, notice where in the body your breath goes. This is breath awareness. It's our porthole into our body and into all the subtle layers of the body. Breath is everything.

Don't worry – you will lose track of your breath and you'll remember five minutes later or five postures later. It doesn't matter. Losing breath awareness doesn't matter. Each time just return to awareness of breath. In time, with this constant cultivation of breath awareness, you will train yourself to be aware of your breathing.

That's the first step.

From breath awareness then arises the ability to respond to the breath. You become aware of your breath and notice you're holding it, so you focus on breathing in and out smoothly and deeply. That's breath response.

You become aware of your breathing and notice that the inhale is forced and tight, but only in backbends. You get curious:

> *'What does that mean?'*
> *'What happens when I back off and don't go as deep into the posture?'*
> *'Can I breathe free and easily on the inhale then?'*

Breath awareness has moved through response and into teaching – yes, your breath has become your teacher. Any disturbance in the breath betrays a disturbance in your mind, body or energy. We hold our breath when we're resisting reality, when we don't want to see something, when we're afraid.
If you hold your breath every time you go into a backbend, ask yourself,

> *'Why are you afraid of bending back?'*
> *'What is it about back-bending that makes you afraid?'*

Follow the thread and perhaps you uncover a fear of vulnerability, a fear of opening up. Learn to bend back with ease, while breathing fully and you'll find that you're able to be vulnerable and open into your emotional life too.

This is the secret of a home yoga practice – you have a teacher.

It's your breath.

It will tell you everything you need to know about how you're experiencing the postures and what it is you need to do in order to move towards ease.

At first, the way your breath speaks to you is like a foreign language. You know it's telling you something, but you don't know what. In time, you learn the language and the response. This is the gift of a home yoga practice. In class we can all too easily rely on the instructions of the teacher to guide us. At home we have to tune into our internal teacher to guide us – the breath.

Once you're connected to your breath, your practice can flow.

Foundations

The second principle of home yoga practice is to bring awareness to your foundation – whatever aspect of the body is touching the ground in your current asana.

Often the feet, sometimes the hands as well or the hands by themselves. Often the sitting bones, sometimes the backs of the legs and the heels, sometimes the spine. Until you learn to levitate, there will always be some part of you making a connection with the ground.

This is your foundation.

Now, what is your relationship to that foundation? Whatever aspect of you is on the ground, either presses or releases into the ground. This grounding action triggers an equal and opposite action from the earth, as she rebounds and sends energy up into our body and holds us aloft.

Think about Standing Pose, or Mountain Pose. As you stand, you extend down through the pelvis, through the leg bones, through the heels and into the ground. We are active as we stand, not just slumping into the earth or the opposite, tensing ourselves away from the earth. There is an active relationship between us and the earth.

The act of grounding into the earth triggers our expansion to the sky, no matter what part of the body is expanding. In Mountain Pose, our feet radiate into the ground and our spine extends up towards the sky. In Wheel Pose, our hands and feet radiate down into the earth and our belly expands up to the sky.

Sometimes the relationship we have with our foundation is one of release and surrender rather than actively grounding. Corpse Pose is a clear example of this.

We allow our bodies to melt into the ground beneath us. Child's Pose is another example. It is a surrender, a dropping down and a letting go.

But in general, most postures call for an active grounding. Even floor backbends like Cobra ask us to ground down through the tops of our feet and thighs, while pressing our hips into the earth. It is this firm foundation that allows our spine to extend and expand into a backbend, lengthening out of our strong foundation.

Which brings us to Principle 3 – Expansion.

Space and Expansion

In every posture you do, there is an expansion of some type occurring. Often, it's an expansion toward the sky, as in Mountain Pose, or Warrior I. This expansion balances the grounding action. In Downward Dog, the hands and feet ground, while the spine extends up towards the sky, taking the pelvis with it. In this lengthening of the pelvis towards the sky, the legs expand and lengthen too, towards the ground.

Sometimes the expansion is in a lateral direction, as in Warrior II. We ground through the feet, sinking the front leg's thigh toward parallel. There is a skyward expansion through the spine, but the release of the pelvis earthward balances it. The extended arms really bring forth the sense of expansion in this posture, as the front of the pelvis, the chest and the arms open out.

In each and every posture – no matter what is going on – there is a relationship to breath, a relationship to the earth and an expression of space and expansion.

This means that you don't need to learn each posture's alignment by rote. You know as you move into the posture and tune into your breath, grounding through your foundation, where to expand and where to find space. It becomes obvious.

When it's not, you can play around and experiment, working with the body this way and that to see and feel where the expansion comes.

The ability to find space and expansion is particularly important if there is any pain or discomfort in the body. For example, if you're doing a backbend like Cobra and feel pinched in the lumbar spine, ask yourself;

'How can I find space and expansion in my lower spine?'

Use the first principles. Breathe into the area, ground your foundation and see what arises. Trust that this act – bringing awareness to the area and breathing into it – will help trigger the body's own natural movement toward openness.

This willingness to explore and trust as you move your body this way and that, experientially like the first yogis, leads us into the next principle – Alignment.

Alignment

Alignment can be the biggest barrier to a home yoga practice because we're afraid we don't know how to correctly align our postures. Here's a small secret that can help.

A-Line-Ment.

A Line.

Things line up.

That's all.

Knees stack right underneath hips and ankles stack right underneath knees: Mountain Pose. Standing forward bends.

Ankles stack under bent knees, shins are perpendicular to the floor: Warrior I. Warrior II. Lunges. Bridge.

Wrists, elbows and shoulders line up: Downward dog. Half Downward Dog. Warrior I. Wheel.

Hands under shoulders: Upward Dog. Cobra. Crow.

Sure, there are always going to be exceptions and variations. Complicated postures break all the rules (or appear to) but you don't need to worry about complicated postures – yet. After all, if you are exploring complicated postures you'll already have a great sense of intuitive alignment and a good teacher to guide you, right?

No, if you're a beginner or almost-beginner or leaving-beginner-status... all you need ask yourself is;

'How could things line up?'

The difficulty is when we begin yoga, it can be hard to sense where we are in space. We don't know that our limbs aren't lined up. As much as you can, look to see.

Look at your lower joints – ankles, knees and hips. Would it be logical for any of them to line up in this posture?

Look at your upper joints – wrists, elbows and shoulders. Would it be logical for any of them to line up in this posture?

If you're not sure, come back to the first three principles. Connect to your breath, find your foundation, create space and expansion and then use your breath to feel along possible 'line-ups' to see what works.

Over time, and with practice, you'll feel it. You'll know. But if you still don't know, take a mental note of the posture and later, after your practice, pull out one of your yoga books, or go on-line, or ask a teacher at the studio... and research it. Find out. Then next time on your mat, play with it.

A mirror can be a useful aid, or a dark window that can reflect. Watching our bodies means we can see what's actually going on and compare it to what we feel is going on. We might *feel* lined up, but the mirror tells us otherwise.

Step by step, bearing in mind that things line up, even total beginners can learn to sense correct alignment from the inside out. Yes, it will take time. Yes, you won't always have alignment right. But it will unfold, and you will get there.

Trust me.

Before we leave alignment: a word on the spine.

Your spine moves from the pelvis. The pelvis is a hinge joint – it hinges over the top of the leg bones. When you do a forward bend, move from the tailbone – extend the tailbone away and behind you. Hinge from the hips, and lengthen the front of your body forward. No reaching the head to the knee (that's the end result of the forward bend, not the aim).

Think length, think extension, think open chest and hinge from the hips. Did I mention that already. Hinge! No bending the spine!

When you first start practicing yoga you may discover that your pelvis doesn't move. That it's locked in place and no hinging is possible.

If that is the case, you don't fold forward. Instead, you lengthen up and away, growing your spine out of the pelvis and breathing space into the hip joints. Only when the pelvis unlocks can you fold forward. But this is not the place for an in-depth lesson on freeing your pelvis. Just wanted to give you a heads up. More on this later.

In the meantime, remember Principle 4 – A-Line-Ment. When in doubt, see if it makes sense to have joints line up. Wrists, elbows, shoulders. Ankles, knees, hips.

Counterposes

When we find our foundation in a posture and expand out of it we are working opposites within the form. We press down into the earth so we can lengthen toward the sky. We release down into the earth so we can fold forward. One informs the other.

So too does the way we sequence postures.

We're always seeking to find balance and harmony within our mind/body. In general, this means that after a backbend we counterpose with a forward bend. We twist one way, we twist the other – and we counter by sitting still and upright for a moment, allowing the effects of the twist to settle.

In general, a counterpose is simpler than the asana that preceded it. It might be as simple as hugging the knees into the chest while lying on the back. It might just mean Child's Pose or even standing in Mountain Pose for a moment or two to allow the body to settle.

If you've just done a powerful forward bend, a counterpose would be a gentle backbend. Sometimes it's so gentle we don't even think of it as asana. But as you go through your practice, pay heed to the effects of the postures on your body, and where necessary – when tension accumulates because of the asana – immediately follow it with a gentle counterpose.

Understanding this principle of counterposing also helps us to sequence our asana practice.

We want to find balance and harmony in the body, which means going through a range of different asana – forward bends, back bends, twists, inversions, balancing poses. Strictly speaking, this kind of mindfulness of balance isn't counterposing, but *awareness* of counterposing helps us to remember to balance our entire sequence.

Curiosity Defines the Yogi

As children, we can be admonished for our natural curiosity, but it's this inborn questioning nature that we want to re-ignite and cultivate in our yoga practice.

Children aren't afraid of what they don't know. Nor are they afraid of looking silly or being a fool. They constantly ask questions. Just ask anyone who has a three or a four year old.

- What's that?
- Where did that come from?
- Why is it like that?
- What is it doing?
- Can I touch it, play with it, move it?

Our relationship to our experience on the yoga mat is the same.

Be curious about everything that is going on and everything that you're experiencing. Not only does curiosity have the added bonus of bringing us into a tight focus on the present moment, but often asking a question is enough to prompt a *different* part of us to find the answer. Maybe the part of us that resides in Atman.

When you start your asana practice, there will be so much you don't know about yoga or about your body, your mind and your emotions. All kinds of things will happen on the mat. Over time, with patience and awareness, you will learn more and more and more about those happenings, and what they mean about your body, mind and emotions. Staying curious helps you to open into this process. It helps you to own this experience. This is yoga!

Let's imagine you're doing a standing forward bend. You're recalling the cues from class and you know that there is something about the legs spiralling this way or that... but you can't remember which way those damn spirals spiral.

Do you think:

> A. *I can't remember the right way to do it, I'll skip this posture.*
>
> B. *I can't remember the right way to do it, I won't worry about that particular cue.*
>
> C. *Now, which way was it again? Do I spiral this way, or that way (moving your legs each way to see which feels right)?*

Often we're trained to respond as A. If we don't know, we skip it or wait until we can find out from someone else. As we evolve we learn to let it go, figuring the answer will eventually come naturally. Finally, we have the confidence and trust in ourselves to experiment and try the legs (or arms, or hands, or whatever) in each possibility and see which one feels right to us.

This is yoga – experientially playing with the body and the breath to see what feels right to us.

And what does feel right?

What is 'right'?

Come back again to the first four principles.

'Right' is where you're connected to your breath, you're aware of your foundation and have an active relationship to the earth through whichever body part is in contact with it. You're expanding either outwards, upwards, or along-wards... or sometimes a combination of many-wards. Right is when things line up and you can feel it. That's 'right'.

When you get curious, and play in a posture, you can feel that the expansion collapses if you move a particular way, or you might notice that either way is fine, but the opening in the body shifts slightly. In that case, what is 'right' depends on what results you want. Curiosity begins to lead us – in the same way the breath leads us – into the practice that is right for us.

Curiosity takes our practice from being something that is externally imposed upon us, to something that internally arises within us. You're turning into a Yogi.

Playing the Edge

When you practice by yourself, you want to hone your ability to feel into your edge and know when you're avoiding being in the difficulty of a posture or pushing beyond your safe limits.

But do you know where your edge is? Or *what* your edge is?

There are three ways we approach our edge, and they map to the three Gunas, or qualities of nature.

The Gunas are an evolving state of nature. We start with Tamas, the heaviest and lowest Guna. We move into Rajas, a lighter, more action-orientated Guna. We end with Sattva, a clear, calm Guna. Another way to describe this evolution of our mind is from Inertia, to Passion, to Purity. I like that way. First we're not moving, then we're carried away with our movement, and finally we're at one with our movement.

How does this relate to 'Playing the Edge'?

In our practice, the edge is the place where we experience discomfort. Not pain – never pain, but discomfort. There is a desire to want to avoid the edge, to move away from it because it feels icky. It takes work and commitment to stay with it. Our state of mind can directly reflect the relationship we're having with our edge.

Here's how.

Tamas is often described as arising from ignorance, and it's marked by heedlessness or laziness.

If this state of mind dominates we won't know where our edge is, or we won't want to go anywhere near it because it's too much work. We're content to allow our body to take the shape of a posture, without internally practicing yoga at all. There is little or sporadic breath awareness and we may be only briefly aware of our foundation or expansion. We're unlikely to be curious, so we never allow our breath to expand our posture toward an uncomfortable place. This quality of mind leads to boredom.

Rajas is more active and this state of mind influences us to go after pleasure. We chase our desires.

In our yoga practice, this state of mind can manifest as discipline because we take pleasure in practicing. Plus we feel good about doing well and achieving. However, the active nature of Rajas can mean we ignore our edge because we're so focused on doing well and pursuing pleasure. We want to attain that backbend or forward bend and so we push ourselves, without heeding the discomfort that's arising and telling us that *here* is where we should stop and breathe, allowing the posture to expand.

Rajas is likely to want to impose it's idea of the ideal posture from without, rather than allow the posture to reveal itself from within. This quality of mind leads to injury.

Sattva is a state of purity, happiness and knowledge. Our action is free from attachment and unaffected by ideas of success and failure.

There is no perfect pose when we're predominantly influenced by Sattva, there is only the perfect pose for us right now. In Sattva, we allow our breath to take us right up to our edge and we feel into the discomfort as it arises, whether the discomfort is arising in our mind, body or emotions.

We stay with our experience, unless the breath tells us we need to back off, in which case we do, with no thought about 'wimping out', or 'giving up'. Instead, we're grounded in the clarity of knowing that each time we come to our mat, each time we come to a posture, we are different and our edge is different. Sattva allows each moment to be as it is. This allows us to truly feel into our edge as an ever-moving, ever-shifting place of discomfort.

When we play our edge, we're also able to discern our predominant quality of mind. We can notice if we're stuck in inertia and can't be bothered. We notice if we want to push push push and get there. We notice if we're tuned in and clear.

Our relationship to our edge reflects our state of mind back to us, and we can choose to shift. We notice we're being lazy and we respond by stepping into the moment through breath awareness and deliberately moving deeper into the posture to find our edge. Or we notice we are pushing through every posture attempting to achieve something, and we choose to back off, find an even breath and dance with our edge instead of bashing it down.

The edge, like our breath, becomes another clear teacher. It's another principle we can rely on to guide us through our practice, even when we think we don't know what we're doing.

Awareness of the edge also helps us to stay present, which is our next Principle.

Staying Present

'Oh no! I forgot to email my boss.'

'What am I going to cook for dinner? '

'My thighs look so fat in this posture!'

Whatever you're thinking... it's not Yoga.

That's ok. Beating yourself up isn't Yoga either. But it's important to remind yourself of this, because it's all too easy to step onto the mat and go through the motions of a practice while continuously carrying on a dialogue in our head. Even when we're practicing pranayama. Even when we're meditating and even when we're chanting. Sometimes, even when I've got a mudra to focus on, a pranayama to do and an asana to hold... my mind is sometimes still an active low thrum of activity beneath it all.

Put the mind away.

Come back to the breath.

Let the thought go.

Come back to the immediate sensations in the physical body right now.

Over and over and over and over and over again.

This is our practice. This is our Yoga. This is why breath, foundation, expansion, curiosity and the edge are so important. It's very difficult to be thinking about the laundry when you've got so many other things to be aware of right now. That's a good thing.

So as you practice, and drift off, come back. Come back, and come back again. That's all you need to do. Over time, with this constant practice of gently focusing the awareness where we want it to be, we train our mind. We cease to be its slave, and instead become its master.

That's the whole point of Yoga. To master the Self, one aspect of which is mind.

Once we have this all sorted, we have the right conditions in place for the next Principle of Home Yoga Practice to naturally arise.

You can't *make* a seed sprout and grow, you have to plant it in fertile ground, water it, and wait for the sun to shine.

So too you can't make yourself surrender to flow. You have to provide it with the right conditions.

Surrendering to Flow

We now know enough to be able to let go.

Connect to your breath, find your foundation, expand and play your edge. Come back to your breath and see where it takes you, follow it. Find your edge and stay with it, dancing on it.

This is surrendering to flow. It's not something that we can do, it's something that arises when the conditions are right.

Surrendering to flow means we let go of what we came to our mat for, and what we think we might do, and instead see what arises. If we start with our usual flow of postures, we may stay with that usual flow, but find that the quality of our flow changes. Instead of directing ourselves through the practice or thinking about what to do next, it just happens of its own accord.

Initially there may be three or ten seconds of flow. Gradually the flow builds up. We hit a state of flow two or three times in one practice. It lasts for longer and longer. Eventually, the act of stepping on to our mat, closing our eyes and tuning into our breath drops us down into flow where our thinking mind let's go and we shift into a deeper state of being.

We're now practicing Yoga.

If at any time we notice we're thinking, or worrying, or doing, or attaining, we gently remind ourselves that it's ok to let go. That we don't need to think or worry or do or attain. We just need to trust the process – to trust our breath, our foundation on the earth below and our expansion into the sky above. We find our edge and stay present. Cultivating these conditions allows flow to arise.

Flow is the state where the mind has become so focused on an object – like our yoga practice – that it merges with it. Patanjali would call it Samadhi. This is bliss.

You can't attain this, bliss comes of its own accord. Let it come.

Persistence or Bloody-Mindedness

If you are not persistent, you will not have a home yoga practice. Without persistence, you will stop practicing.

You will feel guilty when you stop practicing.

You may walk away from your mat for a day, a week, a month, a year or maybe even a decade.

But it doesn't matter. Not if you're persistent. Not if you just get back on. Again, and again, and again.

It's been eight years of home practice for me. I've stopped and started and stopped and started over and over again. But I'm persistent. I know that practicing at home every day makes me a better person, which makes my world a better world. So when I stop, I start again. It's that simple.

Stopped?

Start again. Now.

Patanjali writes about this too, also in Sutra 1.32.

He says:

'The antidote to interruptions to our practice, whatever causes them, is focus.'

Choose something to focus on.

If focus sounds too wishy-washy for you, re-frame it as bloody-mindedness. Be bloody-minded about your practice. It doesn't matter what you're bloody-minded about, only that it keeps you practicing.

So think back to your motivations. Think about your commitment to yourself to practice.

Cultivate persistence.

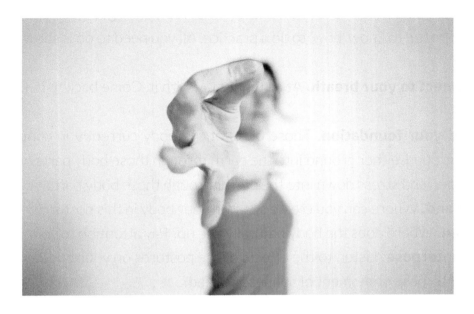

Focus

Conclusion

Those are the principles of Asana Yoga Practice.

When you're practicing asana, if you know and understand those principles inside out, you don't have to know exactly what it is you're going to do on the mat. You don't need to know 'how' to do a practice. All you need to do is show up and:

1. **Connect to your breath.** At all times stay with it. Come back to it. Be aware of it.
2. **Find your foundation.** Those parts of the body currently in contact with the ground, either ground into the earth through those body parts or release tension and stress down into the earth through those body parts.
3. **Expand.** Where can you create space in your body in this posture?
4. **Align.** Where does the body naturally line up? Pay attention to your joints.
5. **Counterpose.** Listen to the effects of the postures on your body. Is a gentle counterpose or moment of stillness needed?
6. **Be curious.** Trust that if you want to know something, you can ask yourself and explore within your body/mind, you will find the answer. Maybe not today, but one day. Just explore and ask and be curious.
7. **Play your edge.** Where is the place in this posture where you are comfortably uncomfortable? Find it, breathe into it, feel it expand. Repeat.
8. **Stay present.** Thinking? Come back to the breath, over and over and over again. Come back to the sensations in the body, over and over and … yes, you know it, over again!
9. **Surrender to flow.** Principles 1 to 6 set the conditions for your practice to arise from within so you can surrender to the flow. Now you're being 'Yoga'd'.
10. **Persist.** Every time you stop practicing, start again. That's all. Start again.

Now you're ready to create your practice and commit to it.

Your Yoga History and Environment

We've broken down the definition of a practice so you know it's not about what you do, but how you do it. We've looked at the obstacles that prevent us from practicing and we've also examined your surface-level and deeper motivations for practicing. We also looked at some basic principles for an asana practice.

It's time to investigate your own personal experience so we can build on our rock solid foundations to develop a practice with a strong framework.

If you've bought this book, I'm assuming you've done some yoga in your life. Usually people don't embark straight into a home yoga practice with no experience at all. Although if you have – good on you! You don't need to have any experience at all to develop and commit to a home yoga practice. All you need is the will to do it.

You've got that right? The will to practice?

Now let's take a look at your yoga history. We're going to get clear on everything that you've ever done before in yoga. Think about classes you've taken, any workshops you've been on, any retreats you've attended, any DVDs you've practiced along with and any home practice you've done. By the way, practicing along to a DVD is not a home practice – it's still externally focused. A home practice is about turning the practice internally.

Think about the teachers you've had, and the styles you've tried. How long you attended something, and why you stopped.

Worksheet 8: Your Yoga History

How you do this is up to you – those that prefer structure can create a table using the following headers and simply fill it in.

Some of you may prefer more creative means, like adopting a timeline or drawing a map. Use whatever process works best for you.

> **Action 1:**
> **Write out your Yoga history.**

Date	Event	Teacher	Style	Notes
2010	Teacher Training	Shiva Rea	Prana Flow	Loved this, expansive & opening. Learned heaps.
2008	Prana Flow Workshop	Twee Merrigan	Prana Flow	My first introduction to Prana Flow – mind blowing. I've come home! This is my practice.
1995	First Yoga	Friend of a friend, Matt	Iyengar	Props, props and more props. I'm still getting into the pose when everyone else is finished!

Allies, Resources and Success

We've already looked at the roles different people play in our lives and talked about the difference between supporters, distracters and naysayers.

Supporters: Help you practice even when you don't want to

Distracters: ,   Help you waver or take you away from your practice

Naysayers: Don't want you to practice

Now let's talk about allies. Allies, like supporters, want you to succeed and will encourage you to practice when you waver or need a pep talk.

The big difference between a supporter and an ally is that you actively recruit an ally and make an agreement with them – so they know what you're doing and exactly how you want them to support you.

Let's say you live with one other person, a good friend of yours who runs regularly. They're likely to support you, and they'd make an awesome ally.

You'd tell this runner friend that you're doing *Forty Days of Yoga*, why you're doing it, what it means to you, and what you'd like them to do to support you.

You can also ask them to follow a contingency plan – if I do this, can you please do that?

- You might ask your running friend to wake you up every morning before they go out for their morning run, so you can get up and practice.
- You might ask them to check in with you every day to see if you've done your practice.
- You might ask them to look after the remote control until you have done your practice.

Beware though, you don't want to turn your ally into a mother or father figure who takes responsibility for making you do your practice – this is handing your power away, and you'll end up resenting your ally.

Part of the agreement needs to focus on what your ally does if you 'kickback'. What happens if they do what you asked them to do, and you get sulky, mad, angry or snarky?

At that point, they have fulfilled their end of the bargain, and need to just say,

'OK. You are in charge of your practice'.

Because you are. Allies play supporting roles, and they're on your side. Don't turn them into the enemy.

The reality is, once you're in the midst of your *Forty Days of Yoga*, and your ally is doing exactly what you've asked them to do, it may conflict with what you want to do in the moment. An ally needs to be strong enough, and compassionate enough to hold the line and stick to the plan. An ally is someone who:

–   Wants to see you succeed
–   Is comfortable standing up to you
–   Has the time and energy to engage with you
–   Cares about you

If you go through your life and can't identify any allies... you need to make new friends. This is when going to a class at a yoga studio, or joining an online yoga community may be valuable.

While we're talking about other yoga students – the best ally of all can be someone who's doing **Forty Days of Yoga** with you. See if you can identify any friends, or yoga students you know who would be interested in working through this book and then doing a forty day yoga practice. Two people on the same practice can support each other to stay with the challenges that will invariably arise. Starting **Forty Days of Yoga** with one or two strong allies on your side is really important. Starting **Forty Days of Yoga** with one or two other yogis ready to go the distance with you: priceless. Topping that, a really supportive studio might run a **Forty Days of Yoga** Home Practice Challenge and invite other yoga students to join up.

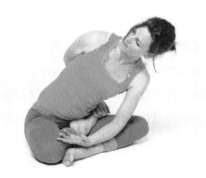

What, or who supports you?

Worksheet 9: Working with Allies

> **Action 1:**
> **Name your Allies.**
> **Make a request of that ally.**
> **Create a contingency plan.**
> **Note any weak points covered.**

Ally	Request	Contingency Plans	Weak Points Covered
Jo – Flatmate	Encourage me each day to practice when you go running.	If I sit down to watch TV at night and haven't practiced, can you remind me of the reasons why I want to complete this sadhana?	Exhaustion at the end of the day when I can't be bothered.

Finding Inspiration and Motivation

There will be times in your *Forty Days of Yoga* when you'll feel low, blah, depressed, exhausted, and so over yoga. Happens to all of us. Knowing it's going to happen means you can plan for when it happens. Those are the moments where you'll need some inspiration and motivation to fire you up.

I've usually got some kind of yoga book beside my bed or in the lounge. When I'm looking for inspiration, I'll pick one of them up. I might only read a page or two, but just diving into a yoga world – especially with an experienced and inspirational teacher – gets me all fired up to practice again.

Some books make me want to try out their specific technique or tool – useful when you're feeling uninspired in your practice. Great yoga books also remind you of why you love yoga, what it does for you, and that it's something worth pursuing daily.

So take a look again at Your Yoga History, and remind yourself of the teachers and styles which really worked for you. Get online, do some research, and see what resources you can gather. If you don't have the income right now to buy more books, or DVDs, go to the library and borrow some. Check out secondhand books. Borrow books from friends. There's always a way, when you've got the will. Collecting fabulous yoga resources is an ongoing quest.

Once you start, you won't want to stop. There's something powerful in surrounding yourself with yoga resources, whether it's books, DVDs, posters, or statues. It's publicly stating that yoga matters to you, that you're interested in it, and that it's worth spending money on. Just seeing these things on a daily basis reminds you of yoga.

That is a fabulous thing.

Worksheet 10: List your Inspiration and Motivation

Action 1:
List the Yoga Resources you own or would like to own.

Resource	Perfect for...
Rodney Yee – Poetry of the Body	Love his dialogues with Nina, plus offers short focused practices I can use in my home practice.
Sharing Sadhana	Great reminder that even successful teachers need to constantly recommit to their practice.
Rumi	Just love his poetry. Love to read a page and then sit and meditate on it.

Past Successes and why they're Great Resources

Just like resources from other people serve as great inspiration and motivators, so too do our own successes.

There have been times in your life when you have said you were going to do something, and you have done it. There have been times in your life when you've done things really, really well. There have been times in your life when you've surprised even yourself at how strong, capable and confident you've been, in the face of adverse circumstances.

Now is the time to remind yourself of all these successes, no matter how little or small they might seem to you.

The purpose of this is to set the psyche up for success. Walking is no big deal right? Just one foot in front of the other. Anyone can do it. Anyone except a baby or a toddler that is. And yet... over time, and with practice, they too learn how to walk. They learn how to balance on two small platforms of skin, bone and muscle. It never occurs to a toddler to give up. It never occurs to a toddler that walking is difficult, or 'not for me'. No, a toddler expects to walk.

It's the same with a home yoga practice. If every other person over the age of 15 had a home yoga practice – even fifteen minutes a day – it would be no big deal. It would be just like walking: a part of growing up and becoming an adult.

Just like walking isn't a big deal, neither is practicing yoga every day – once you get your head out of the way. Toddlers don't have negative self-talk going on in their minds telling them they'll never be able to walk! So let's get *your* head out of the way by setting you up for success.

For some of us, starting this exercise can result in feeling overwhelmed – where do we start? Our lives are littered with success!

That's what happens when you define small successes and look at your life. You see all the great things you do all the time.

Home yoga practice? Just another great thing you're about to do. No big deal.

So the key to this exercise is to just start writing and keep writing.

Worksheet 11: Your Successes

It's important when you fill in this worksheet that you do each action point separately. Don't be tempted to write down one success and then think about the qualities you needed to achieve it. You need to write *all* the successes one after another. This focuses your brain.

The answers will come one after another because there is no thinking required. You're just listing everything you've ever succeeded at.

Here are some prompts if you get stuck:
- What you've won
- What you've created
- What you've graduated from
- Where you've helped out
- What you've been commended for

> **Action 1:**
> **In Column One write down successful event after successful event.**

ONLY once you've exhausted yourself:

> **Action 2:**
> **In Column Two write down the qualities you needed to be successful.**

After you've written down all of your fabulous qualities.

> **Action 3:**
> **In Column Three write down how those qualities will help you complete *Forty Days of Yoga*.**

Success Event	Qualities needed for Success	Useful for *Forty Days of Yoga* because...
Wrote morning pages every day for a month.	Persistence, commitment, dedication	I need to be dedicated to my practice every day, and be persistent when obstacles come up.
Worked two jobs to save for an overseas trip.	Focus, determination, goal setting	I need to stay focused on why I want to practice every day, and stick to my goal of a home yoga practice.

Conclusion

Now you're starting to get an idea of exactly who and what's on your side – you've got Supports and Allies, you've got Inspiration and Motivation and you've got all the Qualities of Success contained within you. There's no question whatsoever that you can do this.

If you want to.

Yep, if you want to. That's the biggest thing. You have to want to turn up to the mat every single day, no matter what. Even when you don't want to. I'll say that again.

You have to want to turn up to your mat even when you don't want to.

How is that possible?

How can You want and you Not-Want?

Easy – there's two of You. There's the You that wants the best for you at all times and knows what you need to do. And there's the you that wants chocolate and wine and can't be bothered and tomorrow is good enough, right? We're back at the Atman (or divine aspect of Self) and the lower Self (the personality with all it's clinging and aversion).

The question is, which You is in the driving seat?

Aligning with Power

Doing an environment scan and coming up with strategies for working with the people in your life is a smart way to keep your practice on track.

Here are a few more smart methods you might want to choose. Not all of these are suitable for all people. Read through and you'll know what methods will keep you coming back to the mat day after day. We all have different Powers – which of these speak to you?

Rewards

You do that, you'll get this. Simple.

If you know you're the kind of person who responds well to rewards, think about what you could do for yourself when you complete your first Forty Days of Yoga. Choose something that you wouldn't do for yourself ordinarily:

Buy yourself something

Take yourself somewhere

Treat yourself to a break

Hire someone to do your housework for the week

Whatever, it doesn't matter. What does matter is taking time to think about what kind of reward would really motivate you to take action.

I'm not much of a big spender – issues with rampant material consumerism and all that – and I've only recently begun to treat myself to beauty treatments.

Like getting a pedicure. Absolute luxury, and makes me feel like a queen for weeks. What about a massage? Divine, absolutely divine. My kind of reward would be to up the ante, and instead of just paying to get my toe nails painted, also get a foot massage and deep soak and whatever else it is they do when you spend ninety minutes with your feet in someone else's hands.

Financially, that kind of reward isn't always possible.

Your reward might revolve around time – giving yourself time to do something that can feel exquisitely indulgent. Like curling up with a good book in front of the fire and reading all day long. It might be something you've been meaning to do for ages and just never got around to – like hiking a spectacular mountain only two hours out of town.

Rewards can also involve other people. You could ask your partner to cook you a special meal. Ask a family member to babysit the children for a night out, or a night in. Maybe you convince your girlfriends to do Forty Days of Yoga too, and all of you go away for the weekend to celebrate.

It doesn't matter. What *matters* is the reward you choose is something you want, but – for whatever reason – have not done for yourself.

If the idea of rewarding yourself for practicing smacks too much of school, or a carrot/stick philosophy, see it as celebration instead. When you finish your Forty Days of Yoga, how will you celebrate? Then it's not that you're doing it for the reward, but that you can't celebrate unless you do it.

Either/or.

Reward/Celebration.

Choose something to mark the occasion. Something you really *really* want.

Star Charts

If you don't like the idea of rewards, you're not going to like my next suggestion. Star Charts. (Or the like).

Bikram and Hot Yoga Studios are fond of using these during their Forty Day Challenges. It's always sad seeing the smiley face stickers petering out for some folk before grinding to a halt well before the finish line. What happened to them? Why did they stop?

They do work though.

Not only will having some kind of chart or calendar on your wall, fridge or mirror help you to remember to practice, it will motivate you to practice. You'll want to stick that sticker, cross that line, or tick that box. Wanting something moves us toward it. Just like wanting to celebrate or wanting a reward makes us more likely to practice.

The fact we're grown adults and could make up as many sticker charts as we like without doing anything at all is irrelevant. We'd know. There's something so satisfying about stickers, lines and ticks.

If you're going to use a chart, make sure you put it somewhere visible – highly visible. Somewhere you'll see it every single morning. This helps to keep your practice top of mind. Things that are top of mind get done. Even if it's just to get them off our mind.

Star Charts, who knew they could be so powerful?

Going Public

Much in alignment with reward, celebration and sticker charts is the public declaration. Nothing like creating external pressure because we're afraid of failing in public, and afraid of what people will think.

Oh I know, we're yogis, we're not supposed to care what other people think and we're not supposed to be afraid either.

But we do care, and we are afraid.

So let's use it.

Before it uses us.

Going public means everyone will ask you how the practice is going. Everyone will know you as that person doing *Forty Days of Yoga*. It means everyone will have something to talk to you about. These are not bad things, although they can be annoying things.

There is something powerful in the group's projected idea of who you are. If everyone around you expects you to be practicing yoga daily, you're more likely to practice yoga daily. Simple. It takes more effort to break free of the Group Expectations than it does to get on your mat. Practicing becomes the norm, the easy option, the only thing to do.

Now, if you're the kind of person that cracks under pressure and shrinks from public exposure, this may not be the right way to motivate you to practice. It could have the opposite effect.

So you need to ask yourself, will going public amp me up, get me excited, make me nervous, make me determined to succeed and show everybody I can do it?

Or, will going public be excruciating, embarrassing, and crush any will I had to practice before I even start?

Be honest now. If you're not a public kind of person, there are other ways to stay on track. Like rewards, celebration, sticker charts and teachers. Yes, Teachers.

Working with a Teacher

I've spent a lot of time in this book emphasizing the importance of a home yoga practice for helping to develop your Inner Teacher. Now I'm going to counter-balanwce that by emphasizing the importance of an external teacher to keep you on track.

We all have blind spots: some of us have blind spots bigger than Australia.

There are things we just can't see, until they're reflected back to us. This is why a mirror can be a valuable asset in practice. We see ourselves in a posture and suddenly realise our left shoulder is higher than our right. We drop the shoulder and from the inside of our body, it feels out of whack, out of alignment. We've been in that misalignment for so long, it feels right.

The same can happen with our mind and our emotions. Unhelpful patterns, negative samskaras, self-sabotage – all so familiar we think they are the norm and we think it's ok.

It takes serious commitment and dedication to notice these ingrained ways of being: but most of all it takes time.

Having an external teacher can jump-start us on this process. An external teacher can see where we're physically holding ourselves, and offer suggestions for ways to practice that will bring us into balance.

Left to our own devices, we're often drawn to those practices which emphasize our strengths and can exacerbate our imbalances. Like Type-A personalities falling in love with Ashtanga or Bikram and using the practice to deepen their Type-A tendencies.

With a good teacher, a Type-A personality can still practice Ashtanga or Bikram, and use those practices to see where they push, push, push instead of gently allowing an unfolding.

A really good external teacher will also be able to suggest practices that not only balance, strengthen and open our bodies, but practices that balance, strengthen and open our minds and our hearts too.

So where do we find such a teacher? Because they are rare. Yoga instructors are a dime a dozen – but yoga teachers not so much.

Here's a few tips:

You want a teacher you can work with on a regular or semi-regular basis, someone local to you and available. Ideally, you'd include a private session every week or two. But if that's not in your budget, then going to class at least once a week with the same teacher and building a relationship that way works well.

Ask other yoga practitioners in your area who they would recommend. In particular, ask teachers the names of their favourite yoga teachers in the area. The teacher's teacher is the one you want to work with.

Don't be impressed with rockstar glamour or put off by quiet, stripped-back teaching. The quality of a teacher has nothing to do with how many students they attract, where they teach, or what they wear. Some of the very best teachers are hidden away in school halls and church supper rooms, teaching a handful of students week in and week out.

Try out at least three different teachers if you can. Start by going to their class and observe how they interact with students. Do they allow students to find their own way to yoga within the structure of the class? Are they kind, compassionate, humble, insightful, smart, and astute?

Find a teacher whose classes work for you. (I'm not going to say 'like' because sometimes we don't like a good teacher's class. It challenges us and makes us feel uncomfortable. Part of us doesn't want anything to do with such a teacher, but the real part of us knows this teacher is good.) Ask that teacher for a one-on-one session. Tell them that you're developing a home yoga practice and would like some support with the process. Be clear on what you want.

A one-on-one session with a good teacher is not just a personal exercise class where they call out the postures and push you through. In a good session, there will usually be some talking at the beginning. Sometimes this talking can go on for fifteen minutes or more. Don't dismiss it, and don't think time is being wasted.

During that discussion a good teacher is noting many things, including your state of mind (Tamas, Rajas, Sattva). They'll note what you believe about yourself and what you believe about yoga. They'll note what's bothering you, what's not working for you, and where you exist in the body. Do you live in the mind? Is your heart open? Are you present? This information will inform the practice the teacher takes you through, and what they suggest you incorporate into your home practice.

After that first session, you go away and you do your practice. Things will come up. You'll have questions. Ideally, you seek answers by yourself, and some of those questions will be answered. But for others, when you go back to your next one-on-one session, you can ask those questions. A good teacher likely won't give you a definitive answer – it's this, or it's that. A good teacher can skillfully extract the answer from you, so you end up answering your own question.

In this way, working with a teacher – although an external force – constantly turns you back in on yourself, reminding you that you know.

A physical example of this: in Cowface pose, when one is sitting on the ground and the legs are wrapped around each other. You might come to your teacher and ask:

Do my thighs roll internally, or externally in this posture? I just don't get it and it feels so uncomfortable.

An instructor would tell you the answer. It's A or it's B.

A teacher would take you into the posture, guiding you to find your breath, your foundation, and the expansion. At this point, the teacher would suggest externally rolling the thighs and ask you what you're experiencing. Where do you feel it? What do you feel? How does it affect your pelvis? Your knees? Your spine?

And again, this time, rolling the thighs internally, How does that feel?

After this guided exploration. You will then *know*.

Not because the teacher told you the answer. But because you were guided to explore and find out for yourself.

That's when working with a teacher really matters, and really works.

A word on cost. Depending on your means, private sessions can be costly. There isn't always the budget for a weekly, fortnightly or even monthly session. But if you value working with a teacher, you will find a way to pay. Look at your budget and see if there's somewhere you can save money to spend on yoga.

Is it worth more to have unlimited yoga classes for a month, or practice at home and have one session with an exceptional teacher? Could you spend less on clothes, shoes, wine, make-up, sports, nights out?

Some teachers are happy to also work for trade. Eg: childcare, housekeeping, admin work, design work.

Whatever it is that you're good at, make an offer. If you can't come up with cash, or trade, and you want to work with a teacher with all your heart... a good teacher would never turn you away.

There's always a way to make it work. *If you want it.* If you have the will.

Ritual

Call this setting the scene. When we do exactly the same things, in the same way, every time, we set the scene for a particular thing to happen. Once those scene-setting actions have been taken, there's no question of the particular thing arising.

That's ritual.

Nothing magical about it. Nothing religious even. It's just that both the world of magic and the world of religion know the power of ritual. It evokes something in us that builds over time.

The ritual you create around your yoga practice is personal to you, and over time, if you do the exact same things in the same order and the same way, day after day after day, you'll create something magical. (Ok, so there is something magical about ritual, but it's not mysterious. It makes perfect sense. Throw the ingredients for a chocolate cake into a bowl, mix and place in the oven, and you're always going to get a chocolate cake. Nothing mysterious about that... but it's a ritual, and it's magical.)

A ritual may be as simple as the way you unfold the mat and smooth it out.

It can be the way you approach the mat and step onto it immediately before practice.

It can be stating an intention before practice.

It can be the way you roll up your mat and put it away.

That's ritual. It's mindful, it's present, it's particular, and it creates a field of awareness for something to happen – in this case, our practice.

Of course, you can make ritual as complex and involved as you like. It can involve candles, altars, statues, flowers, art, music, spaces, invocations, song.

Mostly though, it's just setting the scene and letting yourself know, this is going to happen now.

Like anything, we must be mindful of becoming too attached to our ritual. If we can only practice yoga when we light our special candle and bow to our favourite Rumi poem, we're moving towards dependence not independence. Ritual is about supporting our practice, not suffocating it.

Ritual sends a message too that this is important. That you care about this time, and this practice, because it's worth making special. That means you care about You.

Because you do right?

Music

Adding music to my practice was a major break-through in my home yoga practice.

Actually, it happened the other way around for me. I added practice to my music. A long-time music-lover and avid dancer, I like nothing better than cranking up the dance tunes and dancing it out in the lounge or the kitchen or the hallway. About three years after I'd started a home yoga practice, I found that those spontaneous dance sessions were invariably moving toward yoga, and would go through a natural progression of wild dance, moving yoga, strong standing postures, seated postures, and a closing sequence.

I loved it. It reinvigorated my home practice, and I began putting music on specifically for practice.

But I felt guilty. Real yoga wasn't done to music. Having music on was cheating. It was distracting. It was wrong. That was until I discovered Twee Merrigan and Prana Flow – a style of yoga taught specifically to music. A style of yoga that uses music to induce a bhava (feeling state) and help us drop out of the mind and into the body/heart.

In this approach to Yoga, music was just another tool. Yes!

Even now, loud music invariably takes me to yoga. Putting on my favourite playlists takes me into my practice. Over years of using those playlists and songs to practice to, I've built up positive samskaras around certain songs, especially played in a certain order.

So, if you're a music kind of person, consider using music to motivate you to practice. What helps move you out of your head and into your body? What opens you up? What frees you? I've got a yogi friend who swears by AC/DC, and hey, good on him. If it works for you, it works for you.

In my practice, I use mostly instrumental music, or music with Sanskrit words in it. I'm fond of Kirtan. But there's still those times when I crank Madonna loud to clean house and find myself practicing yoga. Who knew?

Over time, music becomes part of one's ritual. You hit Play and it shifts your consciousness. Just another tool in the toolbox – but a powerful one.

Journaling

Just as ritual signals the importance and sacredness of our practice, so too does taking the time to record our experience.

Journaling – the act of making notes whether words or images or video about our experience – helps us to see patterns and understand the ebb and flow of our practice. Some of us like journaling so much that it encourages us to do our practice so we've got something to write about. Knowing that what we did, whether we did it, and how it was when we did it, is going to be written down makes us more serious, committed and determined about what we're doing.

So there's a two-fold benefit.

First: the ability to see the patterns of our practice and learn from the natural ebbs and flows of enthusiasm, boredom and outright resistance. We might notice things like full moons invariably invoke a more emotional practice where we prefer to slow down and spend more time in seated practices. We might notice that immediately after our moon cycle we've got more energy and want to practice more sun salutations. We might notice that every time we argue with our girlfriend or boyfriend that our practice is fiery and strong.

Secondly: recording our practice makes us feel like someone's watching so we'd better do it (and do a good job) – even though it's just us watching. There's something immensely satisfying about recording something. It's like, 'Yes! Done!' You want to harness that self-satisfaction. Used well, it's a great motivator.

There's many ways you can journal your experience. You could take a photo of yourself in a particular posture every time you practice and see changes over time. You could do a video blog, to publish or not. You could write in a diary. You could record it into your phone. You could use social media and tweet it.

Over time, you're going to build up a wealth of resources that tell you so much about yourself – your body, your mind, your emotions, your moods, the ebbs and flows of You. It helps one get a sense that there is no fixed You, that you are always changing and shifting and letting go and becoming.

If nothing else, before beginning a home yoga practice it can be wise to record what you're practicing, how you feel, what you expect to happen and where you want to go. Later, at the end of Forty Days, (or 400 Days!), you can write again about your experience, results, discoveries and feelings.. Compare the two. There is much to be learned there too.

It's a simple act – to write, to photograph, to record – but it says 'This is important enough to make it part of the written record of my life'.

Which again sends that message that *You* are important. Noticing a theme here?

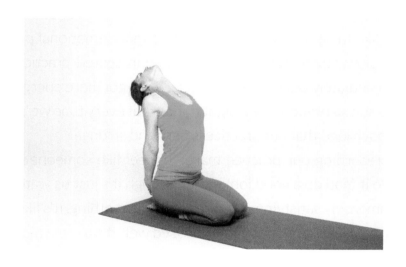

Tuning into Self can provoke insights
you may wish to note down

Worksheet 12: Harness Your Powers

> **Action 1:**
> **What powers are going to work for you?**
> **Cross out the Powers you're not interested in.**
> **Fill in the rest.**

Rewards:

When I finish *Forty Days of Yoga*, I will reward myself...

Star Charts:

I will track my daily yoga practice with...

Going Public:

When I commit to *Forty Days of Yoga*, I will tell people...

Working with a Teacher:

I have found a great teacher to work with –

I plan to work with this teacher in this way...

Ritual:

The ritual I will use to support my daily practice is...

Music:

I will use music in my practice and have organised my yoga music in this way....

Journaling:

I plan to record my experience using.....

Other Power:

 I will...

Creating Your Home Yoga Practice

It's time.

Take all those worksheets that you've already done and gather them beside you. You've dived deep into your psyche and worked out what's really driving you to practice, what's getting in your way, who's there to support you, and who's there to stop you.

You've read and understood the Principles of Asana Practice, and you should have the confidence now to do a practice even though you don't know what to do. It's an important step – trusting yourself and your body to take you through a sequence of asana. Daring to get it wrong and having the courage to explore and play.

You've looked at where you can make time in your day for yoga, and maybe where you can save money for spend on yoga.

You've examined your Yoga History and seen what's worked for you in the past – which styles and teachers made sense to you. In this examining of history you have an idea of where you are on the Home Yoga Practice Evolutionary Scale, so you have guidance on the type of practice that will best support your needs. You also know that we're making up the Home Yoga Practice Evolutionary Scale and you're free to toss it out if it doesn't work for you.

You've lined up your Allies and asked them to support you in your commitment to practice yoga daily, and you've stockpiled inspirational resources for those days when you'll need to get all fired up. You've also looked at your life and seen how many things you've been successful at already, reminding yourself that this success thing is a breeze – all you have to do is show up.

Finally, you've looked at all the different ways you can make your practice more engaging, more enjoyable, and more attractive. You know what you need to do to harness these powers and you've got a reward system lined up, a star chart designed, a way to go public, a teacher on your side, a ritual in mind, a playlist of yoga music or a way to record your experience.

More than anything else you now understand that Yoga is a *how* not a *what*. It's a relationship between things, not the thing itself. It's not asana, it's not pranayama, it's not even meditation – it's a state of being. All those other things, those are tools we use to practice that state of being which is Yoga.

So now, what are you going to practice?

Biggest question of all. Don't be frightened. Let's narrow it down for you.

But before we do: remember this. *What* you practice is not the biggest question of all. What you practice doesn't really matter at all. What matters is that you do something. In the doing, the perfect practice for you will arise over time.

Here's how to narrow down your options. Go back and take a look at the Evolution of Home Yoga Practice. By now, you'll have a clear idea of where you sit on that scale. That's going to answer your biggest question of all:

Do you need a structured practice, or a parameterised practice?

Structured Practice – You know exactly what you're going to do each day. Best for:
- Beginning Home Yogis
- Those who like to be told what to do
- Those who get really nervous and freaked out when they don't know what to do
- Those who wiggle out of anything that's not specific

Suggestions on figuring out what to do:
- Do a one-on-one session with a teacher and ask the teacher to give you a short practice.
- Buy a great yoga book and use a sequence out of that. (Suggestions in the Appendix)
- Buy a great DVD and learn one of its sequences.
- Join an online course and learn one of the sequences from that – like Marianne Elliott's **Thirty Days of Yoga**.

Suggestions of Actual Practice:
-   Five sun salutations. Backbend. Twist. Corpse Pose.
-   Meditate for ten minutes, count your breath up to ten and back down again. Over and over.
-   Alternate Nostril Breathing, nine rounds.
-   Kundalini Kriyas

Parameterised Practice – best for:
-   Yoga teachers
-   Experienced practitioners
-   The highly curious and experiential
-   Those with experience working with mind/ body practices
-   Those with awakened Prana

Suggestions on Parameter Settings:
-   Always set a minimum length of time
-   Be consistent in the mix of asana/pranayama/meditation/chanting

Now, go back and look at what's motivating you to practice – both the surface motivations and the deep motivations.

Choose one, or possibly two of these to work with. Remember this is only for the next Forty Days, and over time you can systematically work through all your motivations. Choose the one that immediately suggests a particular kind of practice for you.

For example, my asana practice usually revolves around my initial motivation for starting yoga – to deal with my chronic back issues. Over time, I've learned how to structure a practice that releases my hips, lengthens my hamstrings, creates space in my spine and therefore releases tension in the back. In practical terms, that means I do a lot of lunge-style postures (Lizard, Warriors), wide-legged squats, wide-legged forward bends, bent-kneed forward bends, and slow mindful backbends.

Don't get too hung up on this process though! Remember, you don't have to get it perfect. It really doesn't matter. What you do on the mat is a small matter.

How you do it is what it's all about. You've got the principles of asana practice to guide you on that one. Although I know for some of you, there won't be any asana in your practice at all.

What does matter is that you open your eyes and you educate yourself on yoga. Let yourself be led. Go to class, read books, watch DVDs. Immerse yourself. Learn what works for you. Experiment. Add in some standing postures. Add meditation at the end. Try a purely chanting practice. Try adding music.

Whatever it is that you decide to do for this first *Forty Days of Yoga*: keep it simple, keep it small.

Better to commit to five sun salutations a day and stick to it, than a ninety-minute practice you abandon in Week Two. Our goal here is to inspire you to practice yoga – in whatever form – every single day. Our goal is not to do a complex practice. Over time – once you have that firm foundation of daily practice – then you can increase the complexity. (Or not).

Worksheet 13: Defining Your Practice

**Action 1:
Fill in this table**

	Structured or Unstructured?
The kind of practice I need:	
The motivation I will work with is:	**Add one or two of your motivations from Worksheet #7 here:**
I will work out what to do by:	
In my practice I will:	**Write a brief summary of your structured practice OR Write out the parameters you'll use**

Creating an Intention

An intention is the foundation of your practice: it's the ground beneath your feet that holds you steady when all else is wavering.

Before we could write our Intention, we needed to do all that investigating of what a home yoga practice truly is, why we don't practice and why we are motivated to practice. Now we have all the background information we need. It's time to distill those pages of information and all the thoughts we've had about them into one simple sentence.

Our Intention.

First, let's get clear on the difference between a results-focused intention and an action-based intention.

We've already talked about why it's important to move away from focusing on the results of our practice and instead focus on the actual experience of the practice. The same is true of our intention.

What makes us turn up to the mat day after day, might initially be the desire to obtain or achieve something. But eventually that carrot won't be enough. We have to actually love being on the mat. We have to enjoy the process and the experience, even when we don't.

It's crucial that when we lay the foundation of our practice – our Intention – that we start with stone and not sand.

Forget about:

'I will touch my toes by Christmas'.
'I will cultivate a calmer state of mind'.

Those are results-focused intentions, and you have no control whatsoever whether or not you achieve those results. You might practice yoga every single day between now and Christmas and never touch your toes. Does that mean you 'failed'? According to your intention: yes, it does.

Here's another way to set an intention.

'I will show up to my mat every single day no matter how I'm feeling or how busy I am.'

Now that's something you can control. Or how about this?

'I will take time every single day to be present with my breath.'

Again, this is something you can control, because it's an experience you can make happen.

That's the power of an action-based intention. You can make it happen.

Plus, you'll notice in our action-based examples above, that one is more specific than the other. In one, we're on our mat. In the other, we're tuning into our breath. The second could mean we're washing the dishes while being aware of our breath. How specific we want to be depends on why we want to practice.

What's the experience we're looking for? That question takes us back to our worksheet on why we want to have a practice. So go back and read through it again, and come back here.

How can you support the experience you want to have on a daily basis by framing it into an intention?

In the example I gave you, the motivation I had for practicing was:

'I want to be able to cope with whatever life throws my way'.

An Intention that supports this might be:

'I will practice yoga every single day no matter what's going on in my life, even if it's just Yoga Nidra before bed, or mindfully breathing through housework.'

This kind of intention gives broad parameters for practice. If I'm mindful of housework, it's practice. This is Karma Yoga.

Your intention may have a tighter focus, reflecting your need to get on an actual mat every day.

This process can be useful to do with a trusted friend, maybe even one of your allies. Sometimes, someone else can read through your motivations for practice and clearly see a great intention for you. Something about perspective and distance. So if you feel stuck, either find someone to help you, or just let it go. You don't have to set your Intention right now. You don't even have to set an Intention before you start your practice, or at all. It might be something that arises for you in the moment, or it might be something that you never need.

As always these are suggested tools.

We're not laying down doctrine here, there's far too much of that in this world as it is.

Take what works for you. Leave the rest, and make sure it is Divine Self doing the choosing, not Ego/Mind self.

Worksheet 14: Setting an Intention

> **Action 1:**
> Write out as many possible intentions as you can.
> Write, write and write until you can't write anymore.

Practice Setting Intentions
I will soften into my practice.
I will follow my breath at all times, honouring it as a teacher.

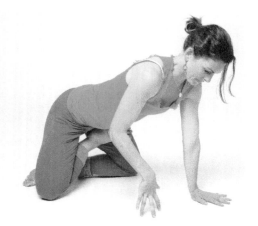

Now we're going to take everything you've done to date and make one final statement.

You're almost ready to begin your *Forty Days of Yoga*.

Worksheet 15: Write Your Practice and Commitment

I, _____, do solemnly declare that I will practice yoga daily for Forty Days in a row, from __/__/__. If I miss a day, I start back at Day One and continue this process until I have practiced yoga for Forty Days in a row.

My Intention is:

My Allies are:

The support they'll give me is:

My Inspirational Support is:

I will reward myself with:

I will track my progress by:

I am going public by:

I am working with:

My daily ritual includes:

My music is:

I will journal using:

My practice is:

Signed:

Dated:

Witnessed by:

Line Up Your Allies, Resources and Support

Don't forget to have someone witness your declaration. It helps to have someone else witness your bold declaration to the world that *this* is what I am going to do. This is it. It might be useful to have one of your allies be that witness as it makes them feel part of the process from the beginning.

Otherwise, call your allies and tell them what you plan to do. Ask for their support. Make sure you're specific. Tell them:

> *'I'm starting Forty Days of Yoga on Saturday and I'm determined to practice yoga every day for forty days. If I do/say such-and-such, can you please remind me of this and this.'*

Get your books, DVDs, podcast, videos and online classes all ready to go. Make them visible – on your bookshelf, your coffee table, beside your bed, beside your mat. Part of this process is setting up your life as if you were a householder yogi, because you are a householder yogi.

Go Public and Start Practicing

Now you've got your signed declaration of practice written out and witnessed, and you've got your allies and resources lined up, it's time to go public.

What did you decide to do?

- Are you emailing your closest friends and family members?
- Telling your work colleagues?
- Facebooking it out?
- Throwing a big launch party for immediate friends and family?

Whatever it was you decided to do... declare it, the day before you start, the day you start, and then if you're brave enough, share progress updates.

Now, you've made it. All that's left to do is... Practice.

The hard work is done. Turning up to the mat will be a breeze. For those days that it's not, you've got the next section of the book to support you. Anytime you need to remind yourself of why you're doing what you're doing, come back to this book and your worksheets. Post them on your wall if you need to. These are your touchstones. They'll keep you on track, hold your hand, give you a kick up the butt when needed and congratulate you when you do it.

You will do it – if you want to.

You want to, right?

That's why you've come all this way.

You want to have a home yoga practice. So do it.

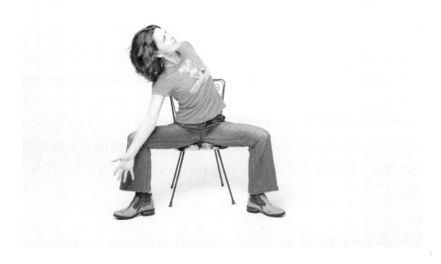

Be creative with your practice –
You'd be amazed at how much yoga you can do on a chair

Sticking to Your Practice: Tips and Tricks

You've done it: you're on your way. The strong foundation and clear-sightedness you've brought to your life, and to understanding your needs, will stand you in good stead as you practice your *Forty Days of Yoga*.

There will be times when things arise that we haven't talked about yet – things like Mat Resistance, Injuries and Illness, Emotional Outpourings, and Failure. There are also conditions of life we haven't yet talked about, like children.

This section of the book gives you tools to deal with all of these, and more.

Mat Resistance: Don't Believe Your Mind

You know you want to practice. You've done all the hard work in making a commitment, but there are still days when you want to do anything but get on that damn mat.

Why not?

I know, you've been here already. You've listed it all out. You know it's a belief in a lack of time, or a belief that you don't know what to do, or a belief in needing the right space first. That's what gets in the way.

But what do all those things have in common? It's not time, nor what to do, nor space that stops you from practicing, it's what you *think* about them.

Your mind: that's the only thing that stops you from practicing yoga every day. Your mind. When you have days with serious mat resistance, it's an aspect of your mind dragging the chain and pulling you back.

Which is why, as you make the commitment to practice daily, you need to keep a close watch on your mind. Don't believe anything it says, unless you have experiential evidence to back it up – and even then – keep questioning it. When that mind of yours throws up thoughts, ideas and beliefs about the way things are, and how these things mean you can't practice – ask it;

'Is that really true?'

Remember, yoga is a journey from the unreal, to the real. When we practice, we learn to watch our mind, we learn to discern what is true and we learn to take action from that place of knowing.

There's even a clearly laid out list of the way the mind can trick and delude us, called the Five Afflictions, or Kleshas. They are:

Avidya – Ignorance

Asmita – I-ness

Raga – Attraction

Dvesha – Aversion

Abhinivesha – Clinging to life and fear of death

You may wonder how on earth those afflictions have anything to do with your yoga practice – or lack there-of.

'I don't know what to do.' Ignorance

'My ankle's twisted, I can't practice.' Ignorance

'Yoga's not my cup of tea. It's just not who I am.' I-ness

'A night out with the girls? Sure... I haven't practiced yet. Oh well.' – Attraction

'I don't feel like practicing today.' – Aversion

There are four erroneous beliefs that give rise to the kleshas:

The belief in the permanence of objects

The belief in the ultimate reality of the body

The belief that our state of suffering is really happiness

The belief that our body, mind and feelings are our true Selves.

This is not the place to go deep into an exploration of the kleshas and what gives rise to them, but it is worth touching on these conceptual maps of reality because this is your current operating system – what you believe to be true about yourself and the world.

You believe that objects are permanent, but viewed through the perspective of time, even mountains aren't permanent.

You believe that the body – this material world – is the ultimate reality – until you experience something beyond.

You believe that the state of being you know as happiness is just that... but once you experience Bliss, you see that what you thought was happiness is actually suffering because it's dependent upon external circumstances to exist.

Most of all, until you practice yoga and touch on that aspect of being which lies *beyond* body, mind and feelings, you still believe that you *are* your body, your mind and your feelings.

You are not. You are something beyond.

Yoga peels back reality so we might see these beliefs – literally see the operating system running our current version of reality. Once you can see your own operating system, you are no longer immersed in it, or controlled by its moods. You notice that you are not your thoughts, that your thoughts are not always true, and the beliefs that give rise to your thoughts are not always true.

This is the beginning of clearsightedness – simply the ability to see what is. We begin to *see* our mind. We see through its delusions. We see through the erroneous beliefs that we've long mistaken for happiness.

It's a long winded explanation – but it's got everything to do with mat resistance. Whenever the mind throws up a reason not to practice we train our first response to be:

'Is this true?'

If you perceive it to be true, ask,

'Does it matter?'

For example:

'I'm too tired to practice.'

Is that true?

'Yes, I am too tired, but I can practice yoga while tired.'

Another example.

'I can't be bothered practicing yoga.'

Is that true?

'Yes, it is true, I can't be bothered.'

Does that matter? Who is the 'I' that 'can't be bothered'? What does, 'can't be bothered' mean?

The practice of questioning the mind and seeing beneath the surface helps us to break the patterns that hold us in bondage and keep us in the dark.

Over time, we learn to discriminate between the voice of the ego and the voice of the Atman. Or the small self and the connected Self. Yoga is the journey home from identifying with self and ego to experiencing oneself as Self and Atman and inquiry – or questioning the mind – is the horse we ride along the path.

Weaken Obstacles: Name Them

While our mind tends to dwell on thoughts and feeling as reasons to avoid practice, like 'can't be bothered' and 'too tired', obstacles are real world events and occasions which exist outside of our selves. Things like:

- travel
- weddings
- honeymoons
- impending work deadlines
- new born babies

These obstacles exist all right, and just as we deal with the mind by calling 'bullshit" on much of what it declares, we use the opposite technique on obstacles. These we name and hold up, bowing down before their greatness, so that we might work around them.

Because let's face it, two weeks in Rarotonga might sound like the ideal place to practice yoga, but is just as likely to lead to lazy days by the pool and dancing nights in the bar.

Heavy workloads can suck every last ounce of energy from us, as can newborn babies.

We need to respect the power of these life events to derail our practice so we can take appropriate action.

Here's a few keys:

Get in Early:

As soon as you identify a potential obstacle in your life – a real-world event that could de-rail your yoga practice, name it.

> *'I've got a stag party all next weekend, it's going to be difficult to practice.'*

Once you've named it, make a plan to deal with it. Work out when, on the days when the obstacle occurs, you can most likely practice.

> *'Golf doesn't start until 9am Saturday morning. If I take it easy the night before, I can do a thirty minute asana practice in the morning while everyone else is still sleeping it off.'*

Now write down what you plan to do and share it with the other people involved in your life these days. Get everything in place that will help you to follow through with your intention and then...

Just Do It:

That's what it always comes down to – just doing it. But it will be much easier to deal with obstacles by naming them, working out a plan, writing it down and sharing it.

Otherwise, you have a big night with the boys on Friday night and wake up late Saturday morning feeling terrible. Your yoga practice goes out the window.

Planning is everything.

Procrastination

Of all the things you'll face that stop you getting on the mat, this is the deadliest.

Procrastination is nothing more than your lower Self fighting your Higher Self. It's the part of you that doesn't want to change, that's afraid of facing truth, feelings and reality, the part of you that sulks and pouts and says,

'I don't want to.'

Deadly.

Procrastination says;

'I'll do it after breakfast.'
'I'll do it at lunchtime.'
'I'll do it after work.'
'I'll do it after dinner.'

Procrastination does anything it can to delay your practice until later. But, later wears out the day and it's tomorrow already.

Here's an antidote for procrastination.

Name it.

Explore it.

Ignore it.

Notice when you're procrastinating and say it aloud or to one of your Allies.

'Oh, I'm procrastinating about doing my practice.'

Take a breath or two and feel into your body. Notice any sensations arising. Where do you feel this procrastination? This is as much a part of your practice as getting on the mat is your practice. It's turning yoga into a tool.

I used to feel procrastination in my belly, and it felt like dread. So why was I dreading my practice? What was so terrible about practicing? Tears. I dreaded crying. Feeling into my body, feeling into the resistance and feeling the underlying nature of the procrastination taught me this. Once I was able to identify and label what was happening, some of the resistance would melt away.

'Oh, I'm dreading the tears that are going to come up on the mat this afternoon.'

By this time, I realised I always felt better after the tears – like a big storm had come and gone leaving a shiny new world in its wake. That meant I could focus on the feelings after the tears. Not the dread, but the relief.

Eventually, this process of feeling into the procrastination turned into motivation.

> *'Oh, I've got serious mat resistance. Serious dread. Must be a big crying session coming up. I'll feel amazing afterward. Woo hoo! Time to get on my mat.'*

I would relish getting on the mat because I knew where I was going.

Most of us are trained to stop at procrastination. We feel it, we hear it, we listen to it.

Break the cycle.

Feel it, hear it, name it, explore it, ignore it.

After a while you will get intimate with the reasons why you procrastinate. You will learn more as layers of the Self reveal themselves. If answers aren't immediately forthcoming when you explore your procrastination, ask lots of questions. You may not 'hear' or 'feel' an answer immediately but over time, answers will arise.

Ask questions like:

- *'What am I afraid of?'*
- *'What am I afraid of happening on the yoga mat?'*
- *'What am I afraid of feeling?'*
- *'What am I afraid of owning up to?'*
- *'What am I afraid of seeing?'*
- *'What am I afraid of knowing?'*
- *'What am I afraid of being?'*
- *'What am I afraid of losing?'*

If procrastination has really got a strong hold on you, make a deal with it. Tell it, ever so sweetly, that you're not even going to roll out your yoga mat, you're just going to lie down in Child's Pose, or Legs up the Wall, or Corpse Pose, and take a rest.

Even procrastination will have trouble saying no to that. When you get down on the floor and into your starting pose, tune into your breath. Feel into your body. Watch your mind. See what arises.

Sometimes, just the act of doing that is enough to calm procrastination and put it at ease so you're able to practice. Sometimes, staying in that one posture is enough for a session.

There were sessions where I'd get into Child's Pose, breath, feel, watch and connect and then the tears would start. I'd be unable to move, unable to go anywhere else.

So there I would stay, for as long as it took for the storm to pass. When it did pass, sometimes I would just turn over and lie in Corpse Pose. That was it. That was my practice. That was enough. Another layer shed. Another truth felt. Another practice of Being.

After a while, procrastination becomes a pointer, a friend, and an ally along the path. It shows you where you're still afraid, and it points you where you need to go.

Remember Your Allies, Inspiration and Resources

There will be days when you will do anything to avoid getting on your mat, and all the inquiry into mind, or facing down of procrastination or strategising around obstacles will just fall flat.

You still won't want to practice.

So don't. Let yourself off the hook and instead, remember your allies, inspiration and resources:

- Phone a friend
- Read a yoga book
- Watch a DVD
- Listen to a podcast
- Let go and be receptive

Nine times out of ten, you'll find yourself wanting to get back on your mat, even if it is just for Child's Pose.

You need to get on to this fast though. A day is only twenty-four hours, and usually only sixteen hours remain when we wake up.

As soon as you feel the dread sludge of Serious Mat Resistance, take action.

If you usually practice in the morning and just can't, take that time to read, watch or listen to one of your inspiring resources instead.

If you usually practice later in the day and feel it dragging on you like a dead weight, call an ally as soon as you can.

Strengthening Your Motivation

Finally, when you hit mat resistance, remember why you're practicing in the first place. Shift your focus from what you don't want – to practice – to what you *do want* – to experience calmness, to relax your body, to free your neck. Spend just a few moments reminding yourself of *that* want, while consciously breathing.

Be soft with yourself.

Be allowing.

Just feel into the Wanting. Feel it in your body. Feel it in your heart. Feel it everywhere you can.

Let that wanting lead you onto your mat.

Your wanting will become your willingness.

What if all this fails you? If strengthening your motivation fails to inspire you, and talking to your Ally fails to inspire you, and your inspirational resources fail to inspire you... if you just don't want to practice.

Then don't.

Don't practice.

Say it aloud to yourself looking in the mirror.

'Today, I will not practice.'

When you consciously decide not to practice, see what happens.

See, it's one thing to avoid and resist our practice, or to 'run out of time' to practice, or to 'forget' to practice.

It's another to be conscious of the avoidance and the resistance and the sneaky tools our ego uses to get around practice like lack of time and forgetting, and to face that head on by saying:

> *'Alright then, I won't practice. I choose not to practice.'*

This conscious choice keeps us in our empowered state of being where we don't allow the circumstances of life to buffet us this way and that way and turn us into victims.

We are no longer a victim of our mind or our feelings either. We make the choice and we own it.

Full awareness of consequences.

If you choose not to practice, your *Forty Days of Yoga* starts over again tomorrow. Own that.

Now what happens?

Here's what might happen.

When you declare a conscious choice *not to practice,* a little voice inside pipes up.

> *'But I want to practice.'*

What?

> *I want to practice?*

You what?

> *'I WANT TO PRACTICE!'*

Really?

You want to practice.

> *'Yes, I want to practice because I've made a commitment and I want to stick to it.'*

> *'I want to practice because I love the calm, clear state of being I experience during and after practice.'*

> *'I want to practice because it tunes me into life and makes me soften and relax.'*

'I want to practice because when I don't my back aches and my neck tightens.

'I want to practice.'

That's what might happen.

All our initial feelings and motivations for practice come flooding back and in the wake of a conscious choice not to practice we end up... practicing.

Funny that, eh?

Home Yoga Practice and Children

It is possible to have a daily home yoga practice and have children. I know this from personal experience.

It is even possible to be a single parent and practice yoga daily.

It is even possible to be a single parent and run a business while practicing yoga at home daily.

It's hard. It takes commitment, persistence, dedication, creativity and the ability to let go of an ideal yoga practice.

My practice is very rarely ninety minutes on a mat. More often, it's seated postures while watching my son play at the lake, or standing postures while pausing on a bridge we're walking over, or standing backbends in the kitchen when I'm washing dishes or cooking.

My practice filters through how I parent, how I'm present and what I do with any precious free time I do have. The moment my son takes an afternoon nap is the moment I sit to meditate.

Practicing around a child means you *have* to make it a priority – it's more important than housework, than TV, or than gossiping on the phone to friends.

The best thing is though, a parent who practices yoga daily is going to find parenting easier. That alone buys you time and makes it all worthwhile.

So, how to practice with children? Here's a few things to consider:

1. Make them aware of how important it is to you

How you approach this will differ depending on the age of your child, but the idea is to share with your child the importance of your yoga practice.

Discuss what your daily practice means to you and why you do it. Talk about when you would like to practice and where. Make it a two-way dialogue as well, so your child can share what your practice means to them, and any ideas or thoughts they might have about your practice.

2. Find boundaries that work for you and your children

Again, this will depend on the age of your child.

- When you do your practice, are you completely off-limits to your child?
- Are you in a different room with the door closed?
- Door open?
- Same room?
- Is the child allowed to crawl around on your mat?

Find a balance between keeping your practice sacrosanct and meeting the needs of the family. Older children are capable of playing by themselves for half an hour at a stretch – you can make it clear you're not to be disturbed unless it's an emergency (Detail what that is. Another child stealing the remote doesn't qualify, a head wound does). Younger children can learn that playing around Daddy is fine, but playing on the yoga mat is not.

Bear in mind that practicing when children are young is a great way to train them to be yoga children – that is, they know you practice yoga, and what it means. They learn that practicing yoga is like brushing your teeth, just something that you do.

3. Make it your priority, plan it into your day. Be creative

If you have to take children to after school sports practices and hang around while they practice, take a mat and practice at the sports field.

Get up earlier.

Make it the first thing you do when: the children go to bed, they go to school, they go to daycare.

Have someone watch the baby for an hour a day so you can practice.

Work with your partner so they watch the kids while you practice.

Whatever you do, realise it's up to you to make your yoga a practice and if you use kids as an excuse for not practicing you're really saying, I'm not making my practice important to me, or I'm not important enough to have this time for myself, or it doesn't matter.

And maybe it doesn't. But at least own up to it. It's never the kids that stop us from practicing,

It's only ever ourselves.

Believe it or not, it's even possible to meditate with our children – even young children. Here's how.

Ten ways to meditate with a young child

1. Establish the possibility in your mind

I know it's possible to meditate with a young child, so I just do it even with my son Samuel. Other mothers I've spoken to about this have said;

> *'Oh I can't meditate because of my child.'*

So true. You can't. Not while you hold that belief. So first up, examine what beliefs you might hold around meditating with a child. Say to yourself:

> *'I effortlessly meditate daily with my child.'*

Notice how it feels in your body, or what thoughts float up in your mind. Any resistance there? What kind of resistance? Can you let it go? Can you establish a new belief? Can you open to the possibility that meditating with a young child is not only possible, but joyful?

2. Start young

If at all possible, get into the routine of meditating with your child when they're first born. God knows you need it! Then they get used to the idea that Mum or Dad sits still and quiet beside them while they play.

3. Be open to the experience

Meditating with a child is a different experience than meditating by yourself. Accept that. Let go of any attachments you have to a completely undisturbed meditation. You will be disturbed, and that's ok. You may not go as 'deep' into meditation and that's ok too.

Be open to the opportunities that arise because of this difference. When you meditate with your child, especially if they're less than two years old, you are holding space for their consciousness too. Your meditation becomes their meditation and they are experiencing stillness and presence through you.

Meditating with your child also means that you can enjoy the simple pleasure of just sitting with your child and being aware of them as tiny conscious beings. It's a delightful gift that can surprise you with its richness.

4. Let go of any expectations

My morning meditation takes about thirty minutes, although when possible, I like to sit for forty-five minutes or an hour. However, sometimes this gets disturbed. My son might need changing or feeding. Sometimes he's asleep when I start, and he wakes up – so I have to fetch him and either delay the end of my meditation, or continue with him around.

Sometimes having him around during my meditation makes it really hard, as I feel my attention being pulled – left and right and all around. Sometimes he won't settle and just needs me to play with him.

Whatever arises in this meditative space, I just let it be. If I can't finish my meditation, so be it. Getting annoyed or upset about meditation is counter-intuitive to the process.

5. Choose a meditation that allows you to sit in awareness

My meditation practice is very simple – once I've gone through some mantra, mudra and pranayama, I sit in awareness just watching all that is and that includes my child.

Meditation doesn't mean I try and block him or the world out. It means that I am aware of everything he is doing, yet I'm not reactive. This gives me the space to be responsive when necessary – at times he'll wander over for a hug or to climb all over me and I'll talk to him, or OM to him. Other times, he may need me to untangle him from a toy, or pick him up from a tumble.

When I'm called upon to respond, I do so, with no drama, nor resistance, nor annoyance. My response is as meditative as my sitting.

6. Set boundaries for other family members

Often we also have partners or older children to consider during our meditation. If at all possible, choose a time when you and your young child are the only people in the house. Choose a room that's not used for living so if anyone does come home, they don't disturb you.

Make sure that you turn the sound off on all phones!

Other family members who are old enough to respond or to set boundaries need to do this for you. But you have to be the one to set the boundary. Make your meditation matter!

7. Start with a child-proof room

Essential!

You need to be in a room that's self-contained and child-friendly.

That means no drawers that open, things they can climb on, or items they can destroy. You can't be getting up off your mat or cushion to pull them away from things all the time.

8. Add a freshly-changed, well-fed and well-rested child

You don't want to have to deal with any of your child's needs while you're meditating, so try and choose a time to meditate when all those needs have recently been met.

In the early morning when I've just changed Samuel, he's never ready for breakfast until much later, and he's always well-rested. Plus he's excited that it's a brand new day and is usually in his best mood of the day.

9. Add favourite toys and refreshments

A child needs something to do, so make sure you have their favourite toys handy. Sometimes it can be wise to have their drink bottle or milk bottle close by, or even a small snack like a packet of raisins.

Having the right toys around, and options for eating or drinking, means you can easily hand them something if they need it, without having to get up and dig around.

10. Make the practice daily and enjoy.

Every single day I meditate. As a result, I reap huge rewards. Which keeps me meditating every single day. It's a constant upward spiral. Plus you will never, ever, ever regret meditating.

'Oh damn, I so wish I hadn't meditated today!'

Never gonna happen!

So just do it.

Enjoy the process. Meditating with a young child is rewarding in so many ways, and I'm really curious to see what happens in our meditation/play practice as Samuel gets older. Maybe he'll naturally join me in mantra, mudra, pranayama and meditation as he gets older: maybe he won't.

Stop, Drop and Practice

This is one of my most effective mantras to ensure that mat resistance doesn't derail my daily yoga practice and it works great around children, or a busy life.

I don't use a yoga mat.

Instead I employ a technique of 'stop, drop and practice' wherever I am and whatever I'm doing.

This works equally well for asana and meditation practice.

Let's look at stop, drop and asana practice first.

A key component to making this work well is being mindful of the clothes you chose to wear.

When you're always wearing comfortable clothing there's nothing to stop you from practicing yoga anytime and anywhere. You never have to stop and get changed.

Yes this is only a small thing. But it's another small thing that can mean the difference between practicing and not practicing.

It's not that difficult to find clothes that you can wear every day AND practice yoga in:

- Jeans stretchy enough for Downward Dogs and seated forward bends.
- Dresses with leggings underneath.
- Yoga pants, with long shirts or short dresses over the top.
- Comfortable shorts and t-shirts tight enough to not end up around your neck in a Downward Dog.

There's very little left in my wardrobe I can't practice yoga in: and that means I can stop and practice anywhere, anyhow.

Yesterday I wore yoga pants and a tunic dress to playgroup with Samuel. While I was sitting on the grass talking to the other mothers and keeping a watchful eye on Samuel playing, I was also moving through some slow seated asana – half-lotus, seated wide-legged forward and side bends and Hero's Pose. It's easy to do this, while breathing mindfully and chatting.

No, it's not a meditative go-deep-inside kind of yoga practice. But it is a loosen-up-the-body and free-the-spine kind of practice.

Later, Samuel jumped on the swing and I discovered I could practice standing postures while pushing him. Forty-five minutes later – yes, my son loves to swing – I had worked my way through Warrior II variations, lunge variations, Triangle, Standing Bow Pose, Standing Half-Lotus and even a few forward bends.

It added an extra element of focus and concentration as I noted how the need to push the swing back and forth impacted on my posture. Afterwards my body felt open and warm and I felt grounded and clear. My son loved being pushed for a long time with a happy Mum.

There's all kinds of ways you can 'stop, drop and practice' in your life.

When you go for a walk, wear yoga-friendly clothing so you can stop and do some asana halfway through the walk. When you come home from work change straight into yoga-friendly clothing so it's easy to practice at any stage during your evening – even if that's sitting on the floor in a breath-connected floor asana while watching TV.

The beauty of 'stop, drop and practice' is that you can creatively work with whatever props are around you and these props can help to open your body in new and interesting ways.

When I walk my son around the boardwalk and we stop on one of the bridges, he often wants to get out of his pushchair and check out the water. I use the railings to support myself in a few forward bends. Sometimes I'll do a full standing series using the bridge. The railings are excellent for working with Warrrior III in a supported manner.

It's the same approach when I'm in the kitchen cooking or washing dishes. I might take a moment to do a supported forward bend using a bench. Or I'll hook my hands onto the inside of the bench and do a supported back bend. There's always added nuances that reveal themselves in postures when we support one part of the body so we can focus on another part of the body.

The 'stop, drop and practice' method also works with meditation.

One Saturday night I was out on the town with a girlfriend. We'd shared some wine with dinner and were now at a live gig. I noticed walking into this bar that I was feeling self-conscious. I could hear my mind chattering away and I had a sense of separation from the scene around me.

Part of me wanted to go and get another drink to stop the mind talk and drop into presence. But I didn't. Instead I brought my attention to my breath and to my senses. I began to meditate while standing in the humming bar listening to the music.

Within minutes I felt myself drop into the present as I relaxed and became part of the scene, surrendering to it's flow and joining my friend on the dance floor.

Other times I've practiced stop, drop and meditate have included breast-feeding, pushing my son on the swings, walking and listening to friends. Waiting is also excellent for stop, drop and meditate. Traffic jams, doctor's offices, the dentist... anywhere you have to wait. Bring yourself into a comfortable seated position, feet flat, spine erect and focus your awareness on your breath and being fully present to everything around you. No one need know. You could be surrounded by people.

These 'stop, drop and practice' techniques are different from being on your mat with a total internal focus. A purist might suggest it's not really yoga, or it's not really a home yoga practice. But there is something powerful about allowing your practice to become an integrated part of your life. It's worked for me. It might work for you.

And that's what we want, right? A home yoga practice that works for us. With or without a mat. With or without our children. With or without our friends. With or without furniture for props.

We want to use what we've got, where we've got it, how we've got it. In doing so, all the barriers coming between us and our practice disappear. Any moment becomes a practice moment.

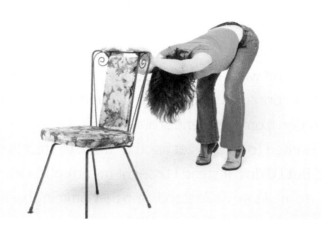

Anywhere, anytime – yoga.

Process:
Dealing with Issues on the Mat

Now that we've covered mat resistance – the things that go on in body, mind and feelings before you get on your mat to practice – let's take a look at what might happen to you on the mat.

Just as it's useful to know what might stop you from practicing, it's also wise to know how to deal with what comes up on the mat: knowing, as always, that other people have been here before. Whatever experience you have, it's not weird, it's not strange, it's just part of the practice.

Missing a Day or Five

Despite all your best intentions, and all your strategies and all your hard work, there will come a day in your practice when you miss a day or five.

It's ok.

It doesn't even matter.

What *does* matter is watching how you talk to yourself about this perceived failure. Watch what demons arise on the inside:

> 'You're no good.'
> 'You never finish anything.'
> 'Who are you to think you can have a daily practice?'

Failure teaches us as much about ourselves as success, and all we're interested in our practice is getting to know ourselves. Yoga is a road back to Self.

So use the experience. Treat it like you would your yoga practice.

When you realise you've missed your practice, take some time to stop and breathe into your body:

- Notice where you feel this missed practice.
- Notice what sensations arise in the body.

– Notice where your attention is drawn.
– Notice what thoughts arise in the mind.
– Notice the quality of those thoughts.
– *Notice.*

As you observe, things will come up. Let those things go. Whatever they are – thoughts, feelings, ideas, beliefs, stories. Oh yes, stories. It is so easy to create a story around an experience. Notice that story and stop telling it.

You missed a day, that's all.

The next day, the day after you missed your yoga practice, get out of bed and practice.

This is now Day One of your *Forty Days of Yoga*. No big deal, no drama, just, Day One. Tomorrow will be Day Two, and the day after that will be Day Three.

If you miss another day, do it all again. Notice, let go, and start again. Again and again and again until you get so damn sick of starting again you just keep going so you don't have to start again.

That's all.

Emotional Outpourings

Expect to cry on your yoga mat. Don't expect to cry on your yoga mat. There are no expectations. But there is a possibility of experience. Knowing it is a possibility helps you to be ok with it when it happens or doesn't happen.

– Some people, while practicing yoga, cry.
– Some people, while practicing yoga, laugh.
– Some people, while practicing yoga, cry a lot.

The practice of yoga removes blockages in our minds and in our bodies. Like blowing up a dam, dissolving those blockages can release tears that were never expressed when we first felt them.

If we're not used to crying or we're not used to feeling our emotions, this can be terrifying. It's likely we still have the same behaviour patterns, or samskaras, that led to the repression of the feelings in the first place, so we're going to do our best to stop from feeling again (which is why we often experience mat resistance, sometimes parading as procrastination).

This is the reason why our yoga practice is so powerful. We've been training ourselves to breathe, to stay, and to feel into sensations. Sure, mostly this sensation has been the stretching of our hamstrings or the release of our butt muscles, but the process that's allowed us to stay with uncomfortable sensations in our physical body will help us stay with uncomfortable sensations in our mental and emotional body – sensations that manifest as feelings.

We're training ourselves to stay present. To be alive. Part of us knows that we're now strong enough to handle all those sensations and feelings that threatened to overwhelm us and drown us when we were younger. Now we're able to notice the sensation, witness what it feels like and watch it go.

Oh, it still takes practice and it could be some time before you're truly comfortable with allowing emotion to arise, express and subside on the mat, but the ground work has been done.

Generally, we don't encounter anything we're not capable of handling. However, if you find that the degree of emotions arising are too difficult for you to handle – as they can be when we've experienced deep trauma like abuse – please find some support. Not just a yoga teacher, but also the appropriate counsellor or therapist.

Sometimes our yoga practice can be so powerful it breaks us wide open, and we need more than just the mat and more than just our breath to put ourselves back together again.

Often, breaking wide open calls for our practice to shift to support us. I remember reading about one yoga teacher who experienced a year of deep grief. She'd lost beloved family members so her practice shifted to Child's Pose and Corpse Pose. She'd get on to her mat, curl up in Child's Pose, and sob. She'd move into Corpse Pose, and feel the sobbing wash away. Over and over and over, every day. This was ok, this was perfect.

Stephen Cope, in his excellent book *Yoga and the Quest for the True Self*, talks about the need to develop both awareness and equanimity in equal measure, otherwise our practice can take us to a place where we feel like we're losing the plot.

'Reality is difficult to bear. There is a good reason why we keep aspects of ourselves hidden. Seeing too clearly, or too soon, can create a dangerous amount of instability in a self that is organised about a certain amount of delusion (which is of course how we're all constructed)... Clear seeing needs the calm abiding Self.'
Stephen Cope, 'Yoga and the Quest for the True Self'

So what is equanimity?

It's the part of us that is most associated with the heart. If clear seeing is sixth chakra, equanimity is fourth chakra. It's a strong sense of centred Self, it's compassion, it's the ability to self-soothe – to be able to take care of ourselves, and mother ourselves.

The practice of Yoga builds our awareness, and when done with loving-kindness and compassion for Self, also builds up equanimity.

Unfortunately, while many of us who dive into practice can be great at motivating ourselves, disciplining ourselves, and doing the hard yards – we're not always so good at being kind to ourselves, or compassionate, or taking care of ourselves. Too often, we can interpret the need for self-soothing or self-care as weakness. We tell ourselves:

> *'It's a cop-out to lie in Child's Pose for ten minutes, instead of pushing through our sun salutations.'*

or

> *'It's weak to only do yoga nidra, instead of our strong asana practice.'*

Watch for this. These statements can be false.

Strong practice leads to strong awareness which can lead to the need to take care of the Self. Just as a child needs both father(ing) and mother(ing), so too does our emerging Self need both.

At times, if it feels like you're being broken wide open, and/or falling to pieces, it can be wise to stop the yoga practice. Yes, stop. It's these moments when having a good teacher or at least a wise yogi friend becomes invaluable.

If you're experiencing emotional outpourings on the mat, or you feel like you're falling to pieces, know that it's normal.

Know that a response may be required. It may indicate the need to change your practice, stop your practice, or get outside support from a therapist. If you're not sure, ask your yoga teacher, or find someone you can talk to about the experience. It's crucial!

Working with Injury or Illness

Just as working with emotional outpourings requires us to build our ability to take care of ourselves, so too does facing injury and/or illness.

In the wake of a broken leg, the flu, or illnesses of the mind such as depression or anxiety, it's important to realise two things:

You can still practice.

Your practice will need to change.

Even if you're in hospital, connected to a drip and relying on breathing apparatus, you can practice yoga. What that yoga looks like will be defined by your limitations. You might be restricted to a simple mindfulness pranayama, such as counting the breath to ten and back, but you're still practicing!

So if you're ill, or injured, instead of thinking:

'I can't practice yoga...'

Reframe your situation in this way:

'I can't do my regular yoga practice. What kind of yoga practice can I do?'

Of course, this shift can bring up all kinds of thoughts and feelings about what a real yoga practice is, and it soon reveals any attachments we might have to our current practice. This is, in and of itself, the investigation of our relationship to yoga and our ideas of what it is – this is our yoga.

In the desire to maintain our practice and deny our mortality, it can be easy during times of illness or injury to push our body too hard. We make ourselves sicker, or we hurt ourselves further.

These are the poles we must navigate between – that of desire to practice and denial of mortality, contrasted with an excuse not to practice because we're laid up and can just slack off. Somewhere, in between slacking and pushing, lies our sweet spot – the place where mindfulness takes us.

If we're not already working with a teacher, dealing with illness or injury is the ideal time to get a skilled practitioner in our corner. Not only do we need to modify our practice to allow for whatever illness or injury we face, but the right teacher will help us craft a practice that will support us in our recovery.

There have been times I've been laid up in bed with the flu, and all I could manage was to listen to yoga nidra. There have been times I've had bulging discs in my lumber spine, and my practice was focused around slow, mindful asana with no deep forward bends or back bends.

Post-childbirth, after an emergency c-section, I spent five weeks unable to do any asana at all, so I turned to seated meditation and yoga nidra to get me through.

No matter what's going on with your body, or your mind, there is always a home yoga practice for you.

Start Practicing

Congratulations! By now you have read everything you need to know about creating your home yoga practice. If you haven't yet done the worksheets, this is the time. Either print them out (using the handy Print Package at the end of this book), or grab a journal, or loose leaf paper and start making your way through the worksheets.

This will take time. In many ways, it is the beginning of your daily practice.

Each day, decide to complete one worksheet until you've done them all.

Make sure you take the actions outlined in each worksheet. For example, when you're working out who your allies are, call them and get them organised to be an ally, with all that requires. When you work through the worksheet on Space, make the space for your yoga practice.

While reading the book has been great, and doing your writing is also great... now it's time for action.

So do what you need to do.

Set up what you need to set up.

And start your practice.

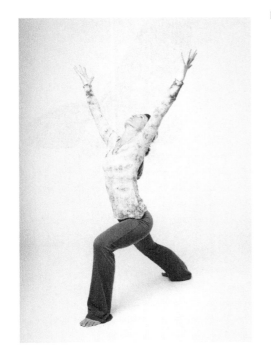

Re-Capping the First Forty Days

Just when you thought it was the end. There's more.

By now, you've either done it. Or you didn't do it.

Or you've done it after a few stops and starts.

How was the experience for you? What did you learn about yourself?

Let's re-cap, and write it down, because it will help you tweak your strategy for next time. There will be a next time right?

This *first* Forty Days; this is just the beginning.

You've proved to yourself that you can practice yoga every day for Forty Days, and that means you can practice yoga Every Day for the Rest of Your Life.

If you want to.

But you don't need to go there right now.

All you need do is commit to the *next* Forty Days.

So before you do, re-cap, learn, tweak, integrate and start again.

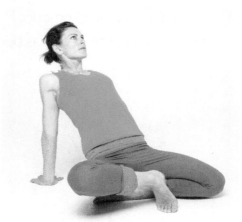

Worksheet 16: Recap

> **Action 1:**
> **Answer these questions**

Did you make it to Forty Days without missing a day?

If you missed a day, why did you not practice on that day?

If you missed a day, how did you feel about missing that day?

If you missed a day, how would you do things differently to make sure you don't miss a day next time?

What was the most surprising thing you learned about yourself?

What was the most challenging aspect of the Forty Days?

What was the most rewarding aspect of the Forty Days?

How have you and your life changed in this Forty Days?

How did your friends and family respond to the Forty Days?

Did your Allies make a difference?

Would you change anything about your Allies?

Did your Inspiration and Resources make a difference?

What would you change about your Inspiration and Resources?

What was the biggest threat to your practice?

What did you, or would you do, to deal with these challenges?

What was your motivation when you started the Forty Days?

Did this motivation change over the Forty Days?

What Powers did you use?

Which Powers really made a difference in helping you stay on track?

Would you change the Powers you used the next time?

Did your mind throw up the same old stories, thought patterns or samskaras? What were they?

Did procrastination teach you anything? What was it?

Did you have any emotional outpourings? What were they? Do you need further support to work with these?

What insights did you have?

How does your body feel now? Any big changes? Any small changes?

> **Action 2:**
> **Go back to the Write It Out worksheet and re-do it,**
> **ready for your second Forty Days of Yoga.**

You're off again! Good luck, practice well, stay present, and be kind.

Resources

Books

These are the books which grace my bookshelf, and I return to them again and again for information and inspiration. This is not an exhaustive list of excellent yoga books by any means, but it makes a great starting point for reference.

Birch, Beryl Bender. *Power Yoga.* **1995.** This is a detailed explanation of a derivative of Ashtanga Yoga, and the foundation of my home practice when I first began.

Birch, Beryl Bender. *Beyond Power Yoga.* **2000.** An expansion on the first book going into more depth on pranayama and meditation, but still with great coverage of asana.

Cope, Stephen. *Yoga and the Quest for the True Self.* **1999.** An excellent resource detailing the psychological process of yoga.

Desikachar, T. K. V. *The Heart of Yoga.* **1995.** A classic, and includes Patanjali's Sutras with a translation and explanation.

Farhi, Donna. *Yoga Mind, Body & Spirit.* **2000.** Donna has a lyrical way of explaining asana as she examines its affects on every system in our body. Beautiful.

Iyenger, B. K. S. *Light on Yoga.* **1966.** Another classic, with photos and explanations for hundreds of asana.

Iyenger, B. K. S. *Yoga The Path to Holistic Health.* **2001.** An excellent reference for crafting a practice for specific health needs, plus detailed explanations for common asana.

Harvey, Andrew and Erickson, Karuna. *Heart Yoga.* **2010.** A devotional journey into the marriage of mysticism and yoga, with set practices like The Joy of Creation. Divine.

Hirschi, Gertrud. *Mudras. Yoga in your Hands.* **2000.** The ultimate resource for mudras. Pictures and explanations plus an indepth look at the hands.

Kappmeier, Kathy Lee and Ambrosini, Diane M. *Instructing Hatha Yoga.* **2006.** Not just for teachers, this book is a gem because it lists variations, modifications and cautions for all the asana included. Includes a DVD.

Khalsa, Shakti Parwha Kaur. *Kundalini Yoga The Flow of Eternal Power.* **1996.** The newest addition to my library, Shakti provides a thorough grounding in all aspects of yogic lifestyle and practice based on the teachings of her guru Yogi Bhajan, Ph.D.

Kornfield, Jack. *A Path with Heart.* **2002.** Technically a Buddhist psychology book, this has helped me to make sense of the emotional and mental process of yoga. A valuable touchstone.

Kornfield, Jack. *The Wise Heart.* **2008.** Builds on *A Path with Heart.*

Stapleton, Don, Ph. D. *Self-Awakening Yoga.* **2004.** Don's personal story of awakening prana and how it's affected his practice. Includes a CD of led practices and the book details many practice explorations.

Whitwell, Mark. *Yoga of Heart.* **2002.** My fellow Kiwi Mark Whitwell explores yoga as a journey of intimacy – with ourselves and with others.

Whitwell, Mark. *The Promise of Love, Sex and Intimacy.* **2012.** Mark's brand new book where he outlines a seven minute practice that he promises will open you up to greater intimacy with Self, life and others.

Yee, Rodney and Zolotow, Nina Yoga. *The Poetry of the Body.* **2002.** A conversation between Nina and Rodney on the essence of yoga, including several detailed home practices organised around themes such as playfulness, falling and being present.

Online Resources

Once you commit to your Forty Days of Yoga, you can enlist the support of an online course and community through the following websites.

Forty Days of Yoga Facebook Page. www.facebook.com/FortyDaysOfYoga
A place to share your experience of the book and your Forty Days of Yoga, plus links to information and resources to support your practice.

The Yoga Lunchbox. theyogalunchbox.co.nz The birthplace of Forty Days of Yoga. Hundreds of articles on making yoga part of your daily life.

Peter Fernando. *A Month of Mindfulness.* monthofmindfulness.info A thirty day meditation course led by the gracious Peter Fernando.

Marianne Elliott. *Thirty Days of Yoga.* www.marianne-elliott.com/30daysofyoga Yoga teacher and author Marianne supports you through the starting of a home practice with daily emails and weekly videos

Acknowledgments

As with any creative project, this one has been a co-creative experience. Thank you to my dear friends Melissa Billington, Mui Leng Goh, Sarah Adams, Tink Stephenson and Alys Titchener.

You all asked the right questions at the right time and those questions gave me the courage to abandon plans to write a *Best of The Yoga Lunchbox* book in the middle of a public fundraising campaign. Your guidance helped me recognise I had an original book in me just waiting to be born and that was where I needed to direct my energy.

Thank you to fellow writer and yoga teacher Marianne Elliott for providing an example of what was possible as I watched her write and publish her book *Zen Under Fire*. Marianne thank you for always being so generous with your support and encouragement, both in my life and in my writing.

My Dad's been on my case for years about writing a book, providing a stellar example as he steadily works away at writing a series of novels. Thanks Dad for being so matter-of-fact and insistent on my talent as a writer. And Mum, thank you for letting Samuel and I come and live with you. It's never easy to live with an adult child, I'm sure! Your generosity created the space and inspiration I needed to tune in, sit down and write.

For years I'd known that a book would come when I could sit down and allow the words to pour on to the page. But I couldn't figure out how to get to the place that would allow the pouring to begin. Slade Roberson with his excellent book *Automatic Author* solved my problem. Thanks to his process, I went from book idea to first draft in less than four weeks. Slade, you rock!

Thank you to Michael Hobbs (Boofa) for his excellent photography. At the time, I didn't have a specific purpose in mind for that photoshoot, but boy did those hundreds of shots become useful in designing this book!

I'm grateful for the time and energy my four beta-readers dedicated to this project. Working with the four of you made the book so much better. Thank you Sara Foley, Helen Clark, Lu Cox and Keile Johns.

To everyone that provided help with the nuts and bolts of the book, I'm so glad I had your expertise to call on. Mui Leng Goh, Alys Titchener, Derek Mead, Jonathan Swan, Yvonne Kerr and Matthew Bartlett, I am so grateful for your editing, proofing and print management work. It's invaluable having fresh sets of eyes willing to painstaking read the text and pick up mistakes I was sure weren't there.

Finally, to my Standard Two teacher Mrs. Logan, who took my stories, written so fast the writing was illegible, and rewrote them. Thank you, thank you, thank you. That kind and generous act of yours always stuck with me. I knew that if a busy teacher took the time to rewrite my childhood scrawl, there was a damn good reason. I always remembered both the speed and ease with which I wrote, and the value you placed on what I'd written. It cemented a knowing that I was a born writer.

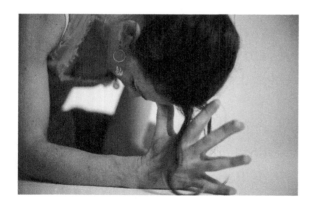

With deep gratitude to the practice and to the divine in me that is also in you.

Kara-Leah, Glenorchy, January 8th, 2013

Blank Worksheets

Worksheet 1: Time

> **Action 1:**
> In Column One write all the possible times you could practice yoga.

> **Action 2:**
> In Column Two write the changes you would need to make in your life.

Possible Times I could Practice	Change I need to make first

Worksheet 2: Places and Spaces to Practice Yoga

> **Action 1:**
> Write all the places you regularly spend time.

> **Action 2:**
> Write all the spaces for each place where you could practice.

Places I spend time	Spaces I could practice

Worksheet 3: Possible Yoga Practices

Action 1:
What do you know about yoga right now?

What I know about Yoga

Worksheet 4: Naysayers and Distracters

Action 1:
Look at the people in your life.
Are they a naysayer or a distractor?

Action 2:
Write at least one strategy per person to minimize the effect
they have on you and your life. Add them to the correct column.

Naysayers	Distracters	Strategies

Worksheet 5: What Stops You From Practicing?

Action 1:
Answer this question.
Why don't you practice yoga at home every day?

Write at least twenty responses to this question in column 2, using a full statement every time. If you start to run out of obstacles, make 'em silly. Make 'em ridiculous. Make 'em up. Get those twenty responses down.

True?	Reasons For Not Practicing

True?	Reasons For Not Practicing

Action 2:
Read each statement out loud and ask yourself, 'Is this true?'
Write True or Untrue in Column 1.

Firstly, let's deal to the statements that aren't true.

If they aren't true then why are they stopping you from practicing yoga?

Because they're an excuse, that's why. So let's answer them. If for example you wrote: 'I don't have enough time in my day.'

You're going to answer with the time you do have, or could make available.

I could get up ten minutes earlier each day and practice.

I could practice as soon as my son goes to childcare for twenty minutes.

I could practice for thirsty minutes as soon as my son goes to bed at 7pm.

Action 3:
Go through all of the untrue statements and write as many answers and as many possibilities as you can.

Untrue Statements	Workarounds

Now let's attend to the statements you wrote that are stopping you from practicing yoga, and that *are* true.

> **Action 4:**
> **Go through all the statements and find work-arounds for them.**

True Statements	Workarounds

Excellent! Now there are no reasons left why you can't practice yoga every day. You're on your way!

Worksheet 6: Building a Yogic Toolbox

Action 1:
In Column One write a list of the challenging situations in your life.

Action 2:
In Column Two write out any yogic solutions you already know about.

Challenging Situation	Possible Yogic Solutions

It doesn't matter if you don't know any yoga solutions – this is just a starting point. Later, you can research and find specific solutions for challenges you face.

This list is something that will grow and expand over time – keep it close and add to it frequently.

Worksheet 7: Assessing Your Yoga Needs

Getting clear on why you need to practice yoga is a powerful process. So is knowing the benefits of a yoga practice, and specifically a home yoga practice. Knowing what your needs are – physical, mental, emotional and spiritual – will help you figure out what to do in your practice.

> **Action 1:**
> **Write down all the physical reasons you need to practice yoga.**

The physical reasons I need to practice yoga

Write and write and write until you can write no more.

Action 2:
Write all the mental reasons you want to practice yoga.

The mental reasons I need to practice yoga

Action 3:
Write the emotional reason why you want to practice yoga.

The emotional reasons I need to practice yoga

The spiritual reasons I need to practice yoga

Whatever, it doesn't matter. The point of this exercise is just to get it all out as if you don't care what anybody thinks, least of all yourself, because you don't. Dig deep, be honest, get silly and write it all down.

Now. Take a break. Go do some yoga. Meditation. Pranayama. Turn some music on. Boogie in the lounge, whatever. Just get out of your head.

Once you've done that, come back and read everything that you're written down – all the reasons why you want to practice yoga. Take a different coloured pen, it doesn't matter. This is your process.

Action 5:
Read through the list and when you get to something important underline it, highlight it, put a star beside it.

Read fast and go with the first instinct. At the end you'll have something like five to ten really important reasons why you want to practice yoga.

> **Action 6:**
> **Write a heading:**
> **My Really Important Reasons for Practicing Yoga.**

> **Action 7:**
> **Read through your underlined highlighted starred answers and tick the ones that leap out at you.**
> **There might be 3 or 4. Draw that many columns.**

> **Action 8:**
> **Write those underlined / highlighted / starred / ticked answers under your heading, one item per column.**

My Really Important Reasons for Practicing Yoga		

These statements are why you want to have a home yoga practice and those reasons 'why' will guide what kind of home yoga practice you do.

In this instance, you may decide to start with Statement 3 and craft a practice that frees up the pelvis, spine and hamstrings so you can tie your shoelaces.

But we're going to take our diving into motivations down another level.

Action 9:
Write those underlined / highlighted / starred / ticked answers under your heading, one item per column.

Your Important Reason	Because – the reason why it's important

It doesn't matter what you write. There are no magic and correct answers here. There are only the answers that you make up. So if it feels like you're making them up, it's because you are!

You should now have a number of important reasons why you want to practice yoga, framed as *'Statement 1 because Answer 1'*.

Action 10:
Take each statement at the top of each column, and underneath write out one sentence in the following format.
'When I *'INSERT ANSWER 1'* it will feel...

Important Reason	Because	I will feel

These endings you've just written are the deeper reasons why you want to do a yoga practice. Not just for getting to the bottom of fear, not just to meet God and not just to tie up shoelaces... but to feel strong and capable, and at one with the Universe. You've now uncovered both your surface motivations and core motivations for wanting a home yoga practice.

Worksheet 8: Your Yoga History

How you do this is up to you – for those that need structure and starters, you can create a table using the following headers and simply fill it in.

Some of you may prefer more creative means, like creating a timeline or drawing a map. Use whatever process works best for you.

> **Action 1:**
> **Write out your Yoga history.**

Date	Event	Teacher	Style	Notes

Worksheet 9: Working with Allies

> **Action 1:**
> Name your Allies.
> Make a request of that ally.
> Create a contingency plan.
> Note any weak points covered.

Ally	Request	Contingency Plans	Weak Points Covered

Worksheet 10: Listing your Inspiration and Motivation

> **Action 1:**
> List the Yoga Resources you own or would like to own.

Resource	Perfect for...

Worksheet 11: Your Successes

It's important when you fill in this worksheet that you do each action point separately. Don't be tempted to write down one success and then think about the qualities you needed to achieve it. You need to write *all* the successes one after another. This gets your brain focused and in the flow.

The answers will come one after another because there is no thinking required. You're just listing everything you've ever succeeded at.

Here's some prompts to help if you get stuck:

- What you've won
- What you've created
- What you've graduated from
- Where you've helped out
- What you've been commended for

> **Action 1:**
> **In Column One write down successful event after successful event.**

ONLY once you've exhausted yourself:

> **Action 2:**
> **In Column Two write down the qualities you needed to be successful.**

After you've written down all of your fabulous qualities.

> **Action 3:**
> **In Column Three write down how those qualities will help you complete *Forty Days of Yoga*.**

Success Event	Qualities needed for Success	Useful for *Forty Days of Yoga* because...

Worksheet 12: Harness Your Powers

Rewards:

When I finish *Forty Days of Yoga*, I will reward myself...

Star Charts:

I will track my daily yoga practice with...

Going Public:

When I commit to *Forty Days of Yoga*, I will tell people...

Working with a Teacher:

I have found a great teacher to work with –

I plan to work with this teacher in this way...

Ritual:

The ritual I will use to support my daily practice is...

Music:

I will use music in my practice and have organised my yoga music in this way....

Journaling:

I plan to record my experience using.....

Other Power:

I will...

Worksheet 13: Defining Your Practice

**Action 1:
Fill in this table.**

	Structured or Unstructured?
The kind of practice I need:	
The motivation I will work with is:	**Add one or two of your motivations from Worksheet #7 here:**
I will work out what to do by:	
In my practice I will:	**Write a brief summary of your structured practice OR Write out the parameters you'll use.**

Worksheet 14: Setting an Intention

Practice Setting Intentions

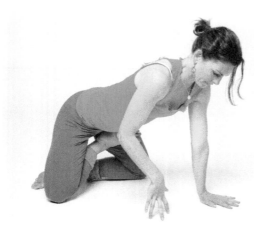

Now we're going to take everything you've done to date and make one final statement.

You're almost ready to begin your *Forty Days of Yoga*.

Worksheet 15: Write Your Practice and Commitment

I, _____, do solemnly declare that I will practice yoga daily for Forty Days in a row, from __/__/__. If I miss a day, I start back at Day One and continue this process until I have practiced yoga for Forty Days in a row.

My Intention is:

My Allies are:

The support they'll give me is:

My Inspirational Support is:

I will reward myself with:

I will track my progress by:

I am going public by:

I am working with:

My daily ritual includes:

My music is:

I will journal using:

My practice is:

Signed:

Dated:

Witnessed by:

Worksheet 16: Recap

Did you make it Forty Days without missing a day?

If you missed a day, why did you not practice on that day?

If you missed a day, how did you feel about missing that day?

If you missed a day, how would you do things differently to make sure you don't miss a day next time?

What was the most surprising thing you learned about yourself?

What was the most challenging aspect of the Forty Days?

What was the most rewarding aspect of the Forty Days?

How have you and your life changed in this Forty Days?

How did your friends and family respond to the Forty Days?

Did your Allies make a difference?

Would you change anything about your Allies?

Did your Inspiration and Resources make a difference?

What would you change about your Inspiration and Resources?

What threatened most to stop you from practicing?

What did you, or would you do, to deal with these challenges?

What was your motivation when you started the Forty Days?

Did this motivation change in the Forty Days?

What Powers did you use?

Which Powers really made a difference in helping you stay on track?

Would you change the Powers you used for next time?

Did your mind throw up the same old stories, thought patterns or samskaras? What were they?

Did procrastination teach you anything? What was it?

Did you have any Emotional Outpourings? What were they? Do you need further support to work with these?

What insights did you have?

How does your body feel now? Any big changes? Any small changes?

Action 2:
Go back to the Write It Out worksheet and re-do it,
ready for your second *Forty Days of Yoga*.

You're off again! Good luck, practice well, stay present, and be kind.

Principles of Asana Practice

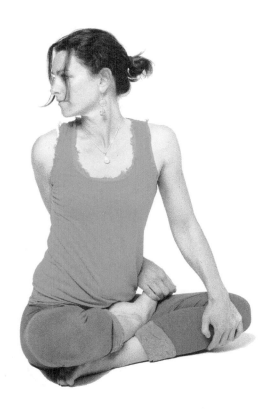

Connect to your breath

Find your foundation

Expand

Align

Counterpose

Be curious

Play your edge

Stay present

Surrender to flow

About the Author

Kara-Leah Grant is a writer and yoga teacher who has always been infinitely curious about the make-up of the human psyche and body. Regular yoga helped her heal and recover from chronic back issues, including a spinal fusion at age 16, two episodes of psychosis at age 29. Her daily home yoga practice began in earnest when people kept asking her to teach them yoga. She's since trained as a teacher with 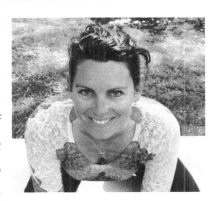 Shiva Rea, and immersed herself in practicing, teaching yoga and writing about yoga. Kara-Leah lives in New Zealand with her son Samuel.

TheYogaLunchbox.co.nz

Karaleah.co.nz

Lightning Source UK Ltd.
Milton Keynes UK
UKOW07f0015170316

270362UK00008B/54/P